Praise for *31½ Essentia*  *Your Medical Practice*

FROM THE FOREWORD BY NEIL BAUM, MD

"Today, many doctors are discouraged about the future of healthcare. I often go to the doctor's lounge or the doctor's dining room only to hear complaints, bickering and overall negativity about what tomorrow may bring. Well, weep no more, because *31½ Essentials for Running Your Medical Practice* is just the book to improve your spirits, improve the morale in your office, show you how to generate new patients, how to develop services that your existing patients need and, ultimately, to increase your bottom line."

NEIL BAUM, MD
Clinical Associate Professor of Urology
Tulane Medical School
Author, *Marketing Your Clinical Practice—Ethically, Effectively, and Economically*

"I can't begin to tell you how beneficial your book is to our Health System. Your chapters on marketing, controlling overhead, and office dynamics have all led to our renewed focus. Our days in AR have dropped significantly, clinical protocol development has improved patient flow and our students are thrilled with the changes in their clinical experience. I thank you for writing *31½ Essentials for Running Your Medical Practice*. In addition to it becoming a valuable tool in the education of our students, it will be a reliable guide for us to provide exceptional patient care."

MARGOT A. SURRIDGE, MA
Executive Vice President & CEO
Rosalind Franklin University of Medicine and Science
North Chicago, IL

"I had the distinct pleasure of reviewing this new text on practice management. It is a great resource for staff members in either a new practice or an established practice. In my more than 40 years of practicing medicine, I have not had a resource as useful as this one. I suggest that every medical practice leader reads this book and put these practical concepts to use."

DR. THOMAS V. MELILLO
President
Ohio College of Podiatric Medicine
Independence, OH

"*31½ Essentials for Running Your Medical Practice* offers a timely and insightful perspective in building a sustainable practice in today's turbulent healthcare marketplace. Pioneers in practice development, Dr. Ornstein and Dr. Guiliana offer accessible business solutions that support quality care outcomes, enhanced patient experiences, and long term financial growth. Traveling North America to give back to their profession and help physicians remember why they went into medicine, Dr. Ornstein and Dr. Guiliana reveal secrets that have enabled them to build clinical centers of excellence and a balanced lifestyle. This is a must read for anyone interested in constructing a successful healthcare practice!"

John A. Romans
President & CEO
BioMedix Vascular Solutions, Inc.
Saint Paul, MN

"In this excellent new book, Drs Ornstein and Guiliana have been able to brilliantly encapsulate the wisdom and knowledge that I have seen them impart in their many live presentations and professional articles. What sets these two men (and this new book) apart are three very distinct points: First, they care passionately about their fellow doctors and work tirelessly to improve their professional and personal lives, second, everything they teach can be applied to virtually any professional practice, and finally, everything in this book is real world and tested, it's not just theory. This new work is destined to become a classic in the practice management literature and it should be on the desk of every professional in North America—as it is on mine right now."

Rem Jackson
President & CEO
Top Practices, LLC
Lititz, PA

"As a state Senator, I have a profound interest in our nation's healthcare delivery system. In addition to the challenges of preventing diseases, treating illnesses, and providing us with a better quality of life, physicians now also face economic challenges as we try to trim down our health care costs. As many industries were forced to do in the past, health care providers will need to continue to deliver the world's best clinical outcomes while still remaining efficient and profitable.

After reading *31½ Essentials for Running Your Medical Practice* it was clear to me that these authors have some answers! This book should be mandatory reading for all prospective, new, and seasoned practitioners. It is written in a clear and concise format, complete with recommendations that doctors can put into place tomorrow. If you are a healthcare provider, you owe it to your patients to read this book!"

Andy Ciesla
New Jersey State Senate 10th District, Assistant Majority Leader
Brick, NJ

"Whether you seek new ways to improve your practice, or face an important management decision for which you need more information, the place to begin your search is with *31½ Essentials for Running Your Medical Practice*. While no book will contain all the information a doctor might need on a specific topic, by simply scanning the Table of Contents of this new book, it is likely that you will find the specific information you are looking for relevant to your situation. You will also find practical recommendations from Drs. Ornstein and Guiliana, two practitioners who have implemented these ideas in their own practices. An outcome of reading this book, that you might not be expecting, is that some of Drs. Ornstein and Guiliana's enthusiasm will rub off on you, inspire you to action, and enable you to have fun during the process."

Jon A. Hultman, DPM, MBA

Author, *Reengineering the Medical Practice: Profit through Efficiency in a Medical Office Environment*

Los Angeles, CA

"Most medical practices struggle to balance all the necessary components of running an efficient and successful practice and marketing is one of these areas that often fall short. After reading, *31½ Essentials to Running Your Medical Practice*, I have made it mandatory that everybody coming through the Integrated MedReps, LLC program read this book. The foundation of a medical practice must be solid to support the growth that all practices strive to achieve. This book reinforces just that, and offers insight and useful information on how to construct and support that essential foundation."

Chad Schwarz

President & CEO

Integrated MedReps, LLC

Morganville, NJ

"As a healthcare educator, I was looking for resources to help train my 32 residents and fellows. When I first picked up this book, I had the notion that I was going to read the same practice management rhetoric that I read in many books and heard at many seminars. WOW . . . I was wrong! Drs. Ornstein and Guiliana, together with Mark Terry, created what I consider to be the "road map to success" for all healthcare providers. Their strategies have made a significant impact on my own practice and patients, and it is now required reading for all of my students, residents and fellows. I also highly recommend it to the attendings. Thanks guys!"

Dr. Ron Guberman

Departmental Director, Residency Education

Wyckoff Heights Medical Center, NY

Armonk, NY

31½ ESSENTIALS

FOR

RUNNING YOUR MEDICAL PRACTICE

BY
Dr. John Guiliana
AND
Dr. Hal Ornstein
WITH
Mark Terry

Copyright © 2011 by Greenbranch Publishing, LLC
ISBN: 978-0-9827055-1-3

Published by Greenbranch Publishing, LLC
PO Box 208
Phoenix, MD 21131
Phone: (800) 933-3711
Fax: (410) 329-1510
Email: info@greenbranch.com
Websites: www.greenbranch.com, www.mpmnetwork.com, ww.mbmbuyersguide.com,
www.soundpractice.net, www.codapedia.com

Greenbranch Publishing books are available at special quantity discounts to use as premiums and sales promotions, or for use in corporate training programs. For more information, please write to the Director of Special Sales, Greenbranch Publishing, PO Box 208, Phoenix, MD 21131 or (800) 933-3711 or info@greenbranch.com.

This publication is designed to provide general medical practice management information and is sold with the understanding that neither the author nor the publisher is engaged in rendering legal, accounting, ethical, or clinical advice. If legal, technological, or other expert advice is required, the services of a competent professional person should be sought.

Printed in the United States of America by United Book Press, Inc. www.unitedbookpress.com

PUBLISHER
Nancy Collins

EDITORIAL ASSISTANT
Jennifer Weiss

BOOK DESIGN
Laura Carter

COPYWRITER
Sarah Herndon

INDEX
Anne Seitz

Dedication

*This book is dedicated to our family, friends, office team, spouses,
children and siblings whose incredible devotion creates most of our life's joy
and has allowed us the time and driven passion to create this important book.
We also dedicate this book to every physician and their support staff who
spend their lives giving to others—living and breathing the last line of our
Hippocratic Oath, "May I always act so as to preserve the finest traditions
of my calling and may I long experience the joy
of healing those who seek my help."*

Acknowledgments

Trying to acknowledge all who have been an integral part of our successes, as well as the lessons that they taught us, is a *monumental* task. There are literally hundreds of individuals who were influential in building and strengthening our knowledge base as we evolved through our gratifying journey of practicing medicine. They have each given us a gift as well as the good fortune of having a passion for practice and people management. We know of no "experts." But we continue to be fortunate enough to be in the trenches with other highly professional and knowledgeable people, each sharing with us their great wisdom so that we may help others to achieve their dreams, passions and aspirations.

We speak often about our blessings and the strong foundation of lessons that our parents worked so hard to set for us. We thank them for teaching us some golden rules to live by, like: "Never forgetting that it's all about people" and "That it is nice to be important but it's more important to be nice." To our Moms and Dads . . . none of life's successes would have been possible without your love, encouragement and countless lessons.

Words are inept at describing our appreciation for our life partners Anna and Stephanie, who unselfishly allow us to be road warriors, spending large amounts of time away from home so that we could follow our passions. They are great mothers, human beings and our very best friends. We are grateful for the understanding of our children Stephen, Justin, Marc, Tyler and Zack, who at times do not have us by their sides but know that we are always there in spirit. Additionally, our other family members, as well as our business partners and office team, often make sacrifices that allow us to promote the science and art of practice management. We sincerely thank each of them.

Our lives are surrounded by other mentors as well, each teaching us valuable lessons much like our parents. We recognize all of these people for their commitment to light our torch and keep it burning, which then allows us to pass on the flame to others. They constantly remind us that we never walk alone in our ambition to extend our hands to others in need, and to let them use our hands as a step to elevate themselves to new levels.

As co-authors we must extend our gratefulness to Mark Terry for his incredible talent as a writer and editor. His positive attitude, motivational nature and deep intellect kept us moving forward and on track throughout the construction of this book. Without his organizational skills and his depth of knowledge in publishing, this book would never have become a reality.

Neil Baum, MD has been a great mentor to us and served as a role model of wisdom and experience in the daunting task of writing a book. We thank Neil for writing the foreword and for always being there for us. You are great friend and a great colleague, Neil!

Our publisher, Nancy Collins, opened the door for the publishing of what will be our first of many books. We sincerely appreciate her confidence and enthusiasm in us. From the very first time that we spoke, we knew our relationship with her would be long and fruitful. We recognized that her passion to help doctors was equal to ours and immediately knew that we found the best publisher; Nancy, your team at Greenbranch Publishing is very gifted and you are blessed to have them by your side.

It has been said that "vision is the art of seeing the invisible." We wish to acknowledge the leadership of the Ohio College of Podiatric Medicine, particularly Dr. Thomas Melillo, Dr. Vincent Hetherington, Dr. David Nicolanti, Mr. Jon Carlson and the Board of Trustees, for having the keen vision to help their students optimize their success by adding a 4-year practice management course to the college's curriculum. We are proud to be part of their faculty!

Lastly, Abraham Maslow's writings teach us about the human needs necessary to survive. When all of the "basic needs" (air, food, love, etc) are satisfied, then . . . and only then . . . are the needs for self-actualization activated.

Maslow describes self-actualization as a person's need to be and do that which the person was "born to do." "A musician must make music, an artist must paint, and a poet must write." These undiscovered needs make themselves felt in signs of restlessness. The person feels on edge, tense, lacking something. In the struggle for the basic needs, if a person is hungry, unsafe or not loved, it is very easy to know what the person is restless about. It is not always clear, however, what a person wants when there is a need for self-actualization. We were both fortunate enough to recognize *exactly* what we "were born to do." Writing this book is a fundamental part of our very own self-actualization. We figured it out. . . . We *must* teach and help others!

Our partnership in this journey is, in and of itself, part of our self-actualization. When one of us fumbles the ball (Yes, we indeed fumble every now and then!), the other is always there to pick it up and get to the end zone to score a touchdown. We are truly blessed to have such a partnership and to have reached the pinnacle of Maslow's theory. We understand ourselves and that WE MUST TEACH . . . and WE MUST HELP OTHERS.

In *The Wizard of Oz*, Dorothy envisioned that somewhere over the rainbow she would find what she was looking for, but soon realized after her incredible journey that all she could ever want was right in her own backyard. Please never forget that you possess all of the brains, courage and heart to achieve your success and, ultimately, what we all deserve . . . inner peace.

JOHN AND HAL

Table of Contents

Acknowledgments · viii

About The Authors · xiii

Foreword by Dr. Neil Baum · xv

Introduction · xvii

ESSENTIAL #1 · **Subspecialties & Your Mission Statement** · 1
Who are you? Who are your patients? And what do they want? Your patient demographics determine the type of practice you run.

ESSENTIAL #2 · **Choosing Your Office Location** · 5
Location . . . location . . . location. How your office location affects your marketing and your practice's success.

ESSENTIAL #3 · **The Business Plan** · 9
Something you can "bank on." Creating the business plan your bank will require and admire.

ESSENTIAL #4 · **Choosing Your Corporate Structure** · 15
The accountant's alphabet soup: C-corp, S-corp, LLC, PC.

ESSENTIAL #5 · **Developing A Budget** · 17
Budget for the first year, budget for every year.

ESSENTIAL #6 · **Hiring Your Staff** · 21
Behind every successful doctor is an efficient staff. How many people should you hire and what skills should they have?

ESSENTIAL #7 · **Leadership Skills** · 27
How to manage your staff and keep your headaches to a minimum.

ESSENTIAL #8 · **Marketing Your Practice, Part I** · 31
Practical steps to getting the patient in the door.

ESSENTIAL #9 · **Marketing Your Practice, Part II** · 35
Internal and external marketing and tracking your efforts.

ESSENTIAL #10 · **Writing Your Office Manual** · 41
What you need to know about your responsibilities as an employer.

| ESSENTIAL #11 | **Office Dynamics: The "EFF" Words** | **45** |
| | Being EFFicient and EFFective with minimum EFFort— developing systems for your practice. | |

| ESSENTIAL #12 | **Motivating Your Staff** | **47** |
| | Inspiration, not perspiration, gets the most out of your employees. | |

| ESSENTIAL #13 | **The Paperless Office** | **51** |
| | Electronic medical records, digital equipment and health information technology. | |

| ESSENTIAL #14 | **Remote Access** | **53** |
| | "I'll have an office—and I'll take it to go." Working from home or on the road. | |

| ESSENTIAL #15 | **E-prescribing** | **57** |
| | Reaping the rewards of e-prescribing systems. | |

| ESSENTIAL #16 | **Billing Company Or In-house Billing?** | **61** |
| | The pros and cons of handling billing yourself or hiring a billing firm. | |

| ESSENTIAL #17 | **Seven Practice Assessments** | **65** |
| | Financial soundness, overhead expenses, managed care costs, patient encounters, services, product, client satisfaction. | |

| ESSENTIAL #18 | **Controlling Overhead** | **69** |
| | Don't get eaten alive! Evaluating and controlling your costs, including salaries, benefits and other expenses. | |

| ESSENTIAL #19 | **Ancillary Services** | **73** |
| | The comprehensive and collaborative care model. Offering physical therapy or other secondary services. | |

| ESSENTIAL #20 | **In-office Dispensing** | **77** |
| | Should you become a product retailer? | |

| ESSENTIAL #21 | **The Art Of Patient Communication And Compliance** | **81** |
| | Getting your patients to say "yes." Presenting your treatment plan and getting patients to follow it. | |

| ESSENTIAL #22 | **Five Steps To Plugging Revenue Leakage** | **85** |
| | Collecting co-pays, evaluating financials regularly, creating benchmarks and asking for your money. Don't assume because it's small you can ignore it. | |

ESSENTIAL #23   **Time Management**   **89**
Get off the gerbil wheel and control your life and practice.

ESSENTIAL #24   **Bringing On An Associate Or Additional Associates**   **93**
How to bring on an associate or partner, and what to
consider before you do.

ESSENTIAL #25   **Non-medical Malpractice Insurance Coverage**   **97**
Malpractice insurance is a given, but what other types
of insurance should your practice have?

ESSENTIAL #26   **Thoughts On Office Design**   **101**
Efficiency, storage and décor.

ESSENTIAL #27   **Dealing With Stress**   **105**
How to make sure your job doesn't kill you.

ESSENTIAL #28   **Effective Patient Scheduling**   **109**
Tips on managing your caseload.

ESSENTIAL #29   **Tips For Collecting Money Owed**   **117**
Dealing with delinquent accounts.

ESSENTIAL #30   **Dealing With The Difficult Patient**   **119**
More tips on effective communication and dealing with
the toughest patients.

ESSENTIAL #31   **Balancing Your Personal And Professional Lives**   **123**
Business might be good, but there's more to life.

ESSENTIAL #31½   **Action Plan**   **127**

Afterword   **131**

Appendix: Benchmarks And Equations   **133**

Index   **137**

About The Authors

John Guiliana, DPM, MS

Dr. John Guiliana is the managing partner of a busy 4-doctor podiatry practice in Hackettstown, New Jersey. He holds a Master's degree in health care management and is a nationally recognized professional speaker and author on medical practice management. Many medical specialties enjoy his frequent seminars on topics germane to practice success. Dr. Guiliana is a Diplomate of the American Board of Podiatric Surgery, a Fellow in the American College of Foot and Ankle Surgeons, and a member of the American Podiatric Medical Association, the American Diabetes Association and the Council on Diabetic Foot Care. He is a frequent contributor to *Podiatry Management* and *Podiatry Today*, and is author of *Talking Practice Enhancement*, an American Podiatric Medical Association monthly news column. In 2006, he was recognized as one of the Most Influential Podiatrists by *Podiatry Management*.

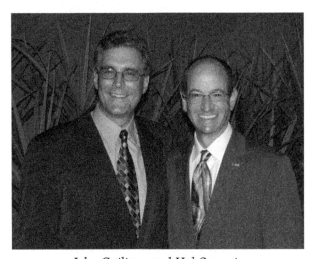

John Guiliana and Hal Ornstein

Hal Ornstein, DPM, FACFAS

Dr. Hal Ornstein proudly serves as Chairman and Director of Corporate Development of the American Academy of Podiatric Practice Management, and Consulting Editor for *Podiatry Management* magazine. Dr. Ornstein developed the 4-year practice management course at the Ohio College of Podiatric Medicine, where he also serves as faculty. He is a Distinguished Practitioner in the National Academies, has given over 250 presentations internationally, and has written and been interviewed for over 300 articles on topics pertinent to practice management, patient satisfaction and efficiency in a medical practice. In 2009, he was inducted into the Podiatric Hall of Fame and received the *Podiatry Management* magazine Lifetime Achievement Award. His personal mission statement is: "Everyday an Opportunity to Create and Share Miles of Smiles." He works to help others change their paradigm to show that "Life Just Gets Better" and to have them define and reach the pinnacle of their success. Dr. Ornstein has been in private practice for over 20 years and serves as Medical Director of Affiliated Foot and Ankle Center, LLP, with their main office in Howell, New Jersey, where he also lives with his amazing wife Anna and 2 lovely boys, Tyler and Zack. Dr. Ornstein also has an office in Edison, Carteret and Monroe, New Jersey and can be contacted at *hornstein@aappm.org* and (732) 905-1110.

Mark Terry

Mark Terry is a freelance writer and editor specializing in the business of health care and physician practice management. In addition to numerous booklength market reports about various aspects of health care, his articles on practice management have appeared in *Podiatry Management*, *Podiatry Online*, *Unique Opportunities*, *Advisor for Medical & Professional Staff Services*, *Veterinary Economics*, *Health Care Weekly—Review* and *Best Practices in Emergency Services*. He is also the author of 8 novels, 2 of which have been translated into Slovak, French and German.

Foreword

Today, many doctors are discouraged about the future of healthcare. I often go to the doctor's lounge or the doctor's dining room only to hear complaints, bickering and overall negativity about what tomorrow may bring. Well, weep no more, because *31½ Essentials for Running Your Medical Practice* is just the book to improve your spirits, improve the morale of your office, show you how to generate new patients, how to develop services that your existing patients need and, ultimately, to increase your bottom line.

Let me explain how this book is written. First, it is not a philosophical discussion about goal setting and being nice to patients (of course, these are important and vital), but provides very specific suggestions that any doctor can easily implement into his/her practice. This book offers 31½ techniques and ideas that have been tested and proven to work not only in Dr. Ornstein and Dr. Guiliana's practices, but also in other practices that have adopted their suggestions and strategies. Certainly, some of the techniques are either known or used in your practice, but I am certain that there will be others that will be new to you and you will want to consider them for your practice.

Drs. Ornstein and Guiliana rise high above the usual psychobabble of other practice management books, leaving theory and tradition in their wake as they alert the medical community to the realities of running a productive and profitable medical practice in the current uncertainties of health care reform.

This book truly offers the nuts and bolts of creating and even sculpting the exact kind of practice that you would like to have. The doctors will teach you how to attract the exact kind of patients that you want. You can tailor your practice to certain demographics, certain disease conditions or certain procedures that you have expertise in and enjoy doing.

They will describe how to run an efficient practice, in which every patient is seen on time and leaves after having a positive experience interacting with you and your staff. After reading this book and implementing their suggestions, your patient satisfaction scores will approach 100%. Of course, you have to survey your patients to obtain this score, and the book will teach you how to conduct inexpensive surveys that you should do on a regular basis.

Your staff will also appreciate your taking the time to read and use this book. The book provides suggestions to raise the level of staff performance, which is vital to the success of any practice. As a result, you will avoid costly turnover and have a staff that enjoys working for you and will sing your praises, to your existing patients and to potential new patients.

This book takes you far, far from the realm of marketing your practice using expensive advertising. This book will show you the techniques of ethical marketing that you can live with and which won't cost you an arm and a leg . . . or a foot, if you are a podiatrist reading this book!

I believe this book is a must-read for all newly minted doctors, as well as for the seasoned doctor who has been in practice for years but wants to create a practice that provides him/herself with more patients, more profit and, finally, more enjoyment.

Bottom line: You don't have to believe all that is written and all that you hear about the demise of American health care. There are wonderful opportunities available for all of us. I suggest you begin by reading *31½ Essentials for Running Your Medical Practice*. I know you will enjoy the journey.

DR. NEIL BAUM
Clinical Associate Professor of Urology
Tulane Medical School
Author of *Marketing Your Clinical Practice—Ethically, Effectively, and Economically*
(Jones and Bartlett)

Introduction

You've picked up this book. You have it in your hands. You've maybe scanned the table of contents, flipped through the pages to see what's inside, and now you've either bought it or are considering buying it.

You must be a physician.

And not just a physician; you're either a physician already in private practice who hopes for some hints on how to maximize profits and smooth out any of your practice's rough edges, or you're considering going into private practice. You might be thinking: "I'm already running a practice; why do I need these sections on getting started?"

A good question, one that we argued about ourselves. And the answer is: Sometimes you have to recreate yourself in order to get better.

Sometimes you have to start back at the beginning to see how you might change things. That's why.

We also believe this book has value to physician partners, medical practice administrators and office managers, and anyone else employed in the medical office. Not only do we discuss focusing your goals and ways to market your practice, but we offer tips on office communication, communicating with patients and ways to keep the office efficient, effective and happy.

We ought to know; we've done it ourselves. Between the two of us, we have almost 50 years in medical practice and as practice management consultants. We have helped dozens of physicians get more bang for their buck, written hundreds of articles on the topic, given hundreds of talks. We have consulted with physicians and businesses on efficiency and management. We have taken courses and earned degrees.

More importantly, we've applied what we learned to our own practices and found out things that work and things that don't.

And we're here to share them.

We want to congratulate you. If you're new to private practice, you've just added a bucketful of new titles: businessperson, business owner, accountant, bill collector, human resources staff, IT manager, boss.

If you've been doing this for a while, you already know how many flaming torches you have in the air and are probably wondering how best to juggle them. We're here to help.

At the end of most chapters, we have provided an Action Step that will take you from theory to practice. In our 31–1/2th chapter, we have collected the Action Steps into a 29-step Action Plan. If you follow the steps in the Action Plan and put them into action, your practice will become more efficient and your bottom line will improve. It worked for us and it will work for you.

Let's get started.

ESSENTIAL #1:

Subspecialties & Your Mission Statement

Who are you? Who are your patients?
And what do they want?
Your patient demographics determine
the type of practice you run.

Opening a practice can be a daunting task: so many questions to ask, so many decisions to make. Where do I get money? Where should I locate my office? How big should it be? How many people should I hire? What do I need to know to hire them? Should I get a partner? How do I get hospital privileges? How many insurance companies should I make arrangements with?

But before we can answer those questions, we need to address the single biggest question you need to ask: Who are you? Before you can decide how well your practice is doing, you need to know what you want your practice to be. If you already have a practice, it's helpful to determine if it's what you *wanted* it to be and what you *expected* it to be.

It also might be a good idea for you to determine if your practice actually *is* what you think it is. You might, for instance, think that you have a successful practice catering primarily to a gerontology base, but if you analyze your records you might discover that half your clients are actually in their 40s or 50s.

So first, let's begin with that old chestnut, Ye Olde Mission Statement.

Yes, yes, we know. Nobody really wants to muck around with anything much more complicated than: *See patients and make a bunch of money.*

But really, that's not enough. Not nearly enough. Creating a reasonable mission statement is akin to the bull's-eye on a target. Sure, you can practice shooting at anything, but a target to aim at focuses your attention.

Your mission statement is your target.

> *"Creating a reasonable mission statement is akin to the bull's-eye*
> *on a target. Sure, you can practice shooting at anything,*
> *but a target to aim at focuses your attention."*

So, what's your target?

How about: *To provide best-in-the-world care to any patient who walks through my door.*

If you're a cardiologist, that could literally be any patient who walks through your door and has a heart. Or a dentist, any patient with teeth; an orthopedic surgeon, any patient with a knee . . . the list goes on and on and gets sillier and sillier. For the proctologist. . . . Okay, never mind.

Although a worthy goal, it's just too general, particularly if you're trying to specialize or emphasize the uniqueness of your practice.

An example, for the endocrinologist: *To provide top-level care for diabetic patients.*

It's of course possible that you will be a generalist, that you are, in fact, that old-fashioned doc, the family practitioner. That's fine, but what do you really want?

To get to that mission statement, answer these questions:

1. What type of patients do I want to see?
2. In 10 years, I hope to be able to:
3. When asked what I do for a living, I answer:
4. What are your goals?
5. What do you do well?
6. What can you do better?
7. What sets your practice apart from others?

It's not quite enough to get just your own feedback, though. If you have employees or partners, you need their input as well. And remember, this is your target, the destination on your practice's roadmap that you're always steering toward. Every decision you make should move you toward that destination.

Here are some examples of mission statements.

From Miami Children's Hospital:

> *To provide excellent family-centered healthcare to children in an academic environment that meets or exceeds the expectations of those we serve and educate. To collaborate with others in our community to improve the health status of children.*

From Snell & Wilmer LLP Law Offices:

> *Our mission is to take a genuine interest in our clients, understand their objectives, and meet or exceed their expectations. We dedicate ourselves to these values: For our clients, we will work hard, provide superior legal services on a timely, effective, and efficient basis, and maintain the highest standards of professional integrity. For our firm, we will foster an enjoyable working environment, based on open communication and mutual respect, and will encourage initiative, innovation, teamwork, and loyalty. For our community, we will continue our long tradition of service and leadership.*

FedEx Corporation:

> *FedEx will produce superior financial returns for shareowners by providing high value-added logistics, transportation and related information services through focused operating companies. Customer requirements will be met in the highest quality manner appropriate to each market segment served. FedEx Corporation will strive to develop mutually rewarding relationships with its employees, partners and suppliers. Safety will be the first consider-*

ation in all operations. Corporate activities will be conducted to the highest ethical and professional standards.

The Walt Disney Company:

The mission of The Walt Disney Company is to be one of the world's leading producers and providers of entertainment and information. Using our portfolio of brands to differentiate our content, services and consumer products, we seek to develop the most creative, innovative and profitable entertainment experiences and related products in the world.

From our own practices:

John Guiliana's:

At Foot Care Associates, P.C., our priority is to deliver quality care to informed patients in a comfortable and convenient setting.

Hal Ornstein's:

We at Affiliated Foot & Ankle Center, LLP are pledged to improve quality of life through treatment of foot and ankle disorders. Our team is committed to a relationship based upon care, concern, and compassion. We will always strive to enjoy what we do.

Now that you have your own mission statement, don't put it in your filing cabinet or away in your desk. Post your mission statement in the lobby for patients to see. Make sure every employee has a copy of it. Include it in the human resources package for every person you hire. Include it in communications with vendors and hospitals you are affiliated with. Use it in your marketing materials.

There's one more thing you need to do with your mission statement and it's by far the most important.

Believe in it. Buy into it. Embrace it.

The mission statement can be addressed on a regular basis and should be, so you know if you're drifting off target. It may, in time, require that you change it. But hopefully, as the years go by, you will discover that your mission statement is a clear representation of who you are and what your practice is.

Action Step: Craft your mission statement. Schedule a 2-hour meeting with your office team to assist in developing your office mission statement, so everyone will have ownership in it. Display it on all written practice materials. Frame and hang your mission statement in your reception area, break room and other key areas.

ESSENTIAL #2:

Choosing Your Office Location

*Location . . . location . . . location. How your office location
affects your marketing and your practice's success.*

It's the real estate mantra: location, location, location.

Picking the site for your practice is not as simple as pointing to a spot on a map. The location of your facility will have a significant impact on your practice.

If you haven't chosen a place to live yet, then where you're going to live and where you're going to work affect each other. If you want to move to Arizona because you want a geriatric population but you hate the desert, rethink your decision.

If you already have a place to live, consider your commute. Not just how long it will take, which is a significant consideration, but the quality of your life if you've tacked an additional 2–3 driving hours onto your day. And anyone who lived and drove through the year 2008, when gasoline prices ranged anywhere from $1.99 per gallon to $4.50 per gallon, should keep in mind that a long, expensive commute can do more than suck up your time; it can suck up your dollars as well.

The first step, once you've chosen a general location, is to study the demographics of the area. But by demographics, we don't mean to just look at the patient population. There are other factors you need to consider.

- How many competing practitioners are there in the area?
- What do those competing practitioners do? How big are their practices? Are their specialties different than yours?
- What are those competing practitioners' ages? This is in case they are considering retiring soon. An area filled with 30-year-old physicians is different than an area filled with 70-year-old physicians.

Calculate a ratio. For podiatrists, for example, we like to see 1 podiatrist for every 25,000 people in the population. For each specialty, your medical association should have recommended benchmarks.

Now, look at the patient demographics. Figure out not only who lives in the area, but who works in the area. Are there factories? Retail businesses? Professional offices? Schools? Universities?

Who's the biggest employer in the area?

Knowing these things will not only inform where you place your practice, but how you design your space. It will inform how many people you hire, the equipment you buy or lease, and how much money you will need to start up the practice.

Sources for this information can typically be found at the local chamber of commerce. If you have plans to work with a specific hospital in the area, they should be able to provide you with useful demographic information.

The Internet can be a source of valuable information; however, as with all things on the Internet, double-check to make sure the sources are current and reliable.

Another important thing to look for is whether the area is growing. An area whose population is dwindling might be a risk.

Also, study the area to see if there are ancillary services to your practice, such as a physical therapy center.

Another factor is to consider what is available in the area in terms of zoned space. Are there houses that you can rent or buy that would be appropriate for your practice? What type of neighborhood are they in? Is there parking? The same goes for storefronts or stand-alone facilities. Where are they in the locale? What's nearby? What is parking like? Access? Good neighborhoods or bad?

If you have those answers, it's time to think about whether you should rent/lease or build your own practice.

LANDLORDS & TENANTS

Before you set up your practice, you need to decide whether to rent or lease space or build your own. Most likely, if you're starting out, the decision has been made for you, because you simply can't afford to build an office.

Nonetheless, let's address some of the issues that crop up for both scenarios.

Renting

Pros
- Typically, when renting, you often need the first and last month's rent, but you don't need a down payment. If start-up cash is an issue, then this is a big deal.
- When you rent, you can pretty much pick the space and size you need. If you start a practice small and expect to grow, this is easier to handle than building, say, 10,000 square feet of space and only using 4,000, but paying for the full 10,000.
- Relative flexibility. If you rent, once your lease is up, you can move if the location isn't working out or the neighborhood has changed for the worse. This is a tough nut to crack if you've built a building.
- Location, location, location: Lease sites often have high-visibility locations, such as shopping centers, that can be difficult to duplicate for property you're building.
- Leasing might be cheaper.

Cons
- Well, you're renting. You don't create equity in your property, your landlord does.

- Any improvements you make to the property revert to the landlord at the end of the lease.
- You have no control over common area maintenance fees if they are included as part of the cost of the lease.
- When you decide to sell your practice, this can become more complicated because the lease may need to be renegotiated or the landlord may need to approve the practice's new owner.
- Expanding the facility may not be possible.
- The landlord may place limits on what services you can offer.

Owning

Pros

- Owning builds equity. The building itself can be a good investment.
- You have more control over expansion.
- It can help fund retirement plans either through a full-out sale or by holding on to the building and renting it to the new tenants.
- If you're actually building the building vs buying an existing structure, you have more control over space utilization and aesthetic issues.
- Owning the facility can make the practice more marketable in the future, by having stability and control over the space.

Cons

- Typically will require a down payment and you pay for the financing.
- If you own a single-use facility, it may be harder to sell as such when the time comes.
- Although there are probably worse things to have happen to you, if your facility's location goes through a real estate boom, the increased value of the property may make it difficult to sell in addition to the practice along with it.
- Local zoning regulations may limit where you can build and what type of services you can offer.

But before you sign the lease or contract, exactly how much space do you need?

FEELING THE SQUEEZE

All this talk of renting or owning your facility begs the real question—how much space do you actually need?

The answer to that question depends on the type of practice you're planning to have, whether you have partners and whether you need a surgical suite.

Rule of thumb: 1,200–1,500 square feet for the first physician; add 1,000–1,200 square feet for each additional physician, up to 4 or 5 physicians. A traditional 1-physician office would have 3 exam rooms, a consultation room, a reception room, and a business office and/or storage space.

So, how big should your reception room be? If you have more exam rooms, you can have a smaller reception room. To calculate, consider your busiest hour and figure the number of patients you expect to see during that time period. Multiply that number by 2.5. This accounts not just for patients, but parents of children or relatives and friends who may accompany the patient. Subtract the number of exam rooms. This gives you the number of chairs.

> *"Rule of thumb: 1,200–1,500 square feet for the first physician;*
> *add 1,000–1,200 square feet for each additional physician,*
> *up to 4 or 5 physicians."*

For example, 10 patients × 2.5 = 25–3 exam rooms = 22 chairs. Crazy, huh? If you're a 1-physician office, you won't be able to handle 10 patients per hour anyway, more like 5 or 6, but there's the math.

Multiply the number of chairs by 20 square feet. 22 chairs × 20 square feet = 240 square feet for your reception room. When designing the space, take into consideration workflow, lunch and break areas for staff and, above all, storage. Going heavy on electronic health records and computers can cut down on storage issues, but not eliminate them.

Also remember: Employees who are walking are not working. Lay out your office for everyone's convenience.

Action Step: List the benefits of your current location (or future office site) and how those benefits will be used in your strategic plan. If you plan to move to a new location or start in practice, list the pros and cons of locations you are considering.

ESSENTIAL #3:

The Business Plan

Something you can "bank on."
Creating the business plan your bank will require and admire.

It is possible to walk into a bank without any business plan or documentation and ask for money. If you're a physician, the diploma itself will provide a certain degree of confidence on the part of the loan officer.

However, that's not really recommended. Better to plan ahead.

That requires a business plan and some idea of how much money you want and what you want it for.

An excellent resource for this is the U.S. Small Business Administration, whose Web site is *www.sba.gov*.

First, there are 4 questions you should ask yourself.

1. What service or product does your business provide, and what needs does it fill?
2. Who are the potential customers for your product or service, and why will they purchase it from you?
3. How will you reach your potential customers?
4. Where will you get the financial resources to start your business?

This is all about identifying your goals, knowing who your target population is and how you're going to serve them. With that knowledge in hand, you should be able to project your potential earnings through your first 3 years of practice. You're going to need to incorporate a marketing plan, so the bank or lending institution can see how the target population is going to hear about you.

A typical business plan has 4 elements. They are:

1. Description of the business
2. Marketing
3. Finances
4. Management

DESCRIPTION

Luckily, if you've already worked through your mission statement, you're almost there with a description of your business. In the case of a business description, you should focus more on some of the nuts-and-bolts aspects of the business. It might be described as:

To run a single-practitioner orthopedic surgery practice focusing on sports and athletic medicine.

It's also a good idea to include your CV, or even just a paragraph or 2 on how you plan to fulfill the proposal.

Additional questions that might come up in your business description:

1. Am I practicing by myself?
2. Am I planning on forming a partnership?
3. Who am I serving?
4. What's my target?
5. Is there competition in the area?
6. What do I bring to the table if there is competition in the area?

MARKETING

Marketing can take on a life of its own and will be dealt with in greater detail later in the book, but, for this section, you should be able to provide an outline of things you intend to do, such as:

- Create a Web site.
- If you're comfortable with it, take part in various social media, such as Facebook and Twitter, although both should come with a warning label that says: Be Cautious, Subject to Abuse. Create guidelines for their use and make sure they're followed.
- Make sure you're listed in professional networking sites like Plaxo and LinkedIn.
- Run an ad in the Yellow Pages.
- Visit local physicians and introduce yourself as a potential referral physician.
- Depending on your practice's focus, visit sporting events, nursing homes or any other place where your patients might be present.
- If you have a relationship with a hospital, they can help with marketing.
- Pharmaceutical vendors / representatives can sometimes help with marketing.
- Send out flyers.
- Advertise in your local newspaper.
- Have an open house (which you will also have to market for).

FINANCES

In a start-up, there are 2 components to your proposed budget: Your personal budget—in other words, how much money you need to live on while your practice gets on its feet—and the budget you set for your office.

Typically, when you're budgeting for a start-up, you need about 6 months of working capital for both your business and personal budget.

The personal budget is fairly straightforward: How much money do you need to live on for 6 months? Include rent or mortgage, taxes, insurance, food, etc. Be generous; you'd rather have too much than not enough.

The business budget can get complicated in a hurry, because it will force you to make a lot of decisions about the type of practice you plan to have. For instance, if you require a surgery suite, you will need a larger space and a bigger budget for staffing and equipment.

The number of staff you need, how much you plan to pay them and what kind of benefits you expect to provide for them affects the budget. Those are big items.

No less important but not quite as expensive are decisions that need to be made about how your office will run. Will you have an answering machine vs an answering service? Will you use digital and electronic health records? Even if you don't have vendors in mind, you need to start making those decisions in order to rough out a budget to take to the bank. This is where hiring a practice management consultant can be very useful, because they can provide a detailed list of considerations and how much they cost.

The biggest trick, at this stage of a start-up, is being both specific and general. You need to create a pro forma budget with estimated expenses and income for the first year of your practice and possibly for 2–5 years. Your guesses will be educated guesses, but guesses nonetheless.

The rule of thumb for your budget for benefits is typically 14%–15% of your budget.

Different specialties' professional organizations often have data available on income, expenses and fees. The Medical Group Management Association's Web site, *www.mgma.com*, has very useful data. There are a plethora of these organizations, such as the American Association of Orthopaedic Executives (*www.aaoe.net*), the American Osteopathic Association (*www.osteopathic.org*), the American Optometric Association (*www.aoa.org*), the Association of Dermatology Administrators/Managers (*www.ada-m.org*), Neurosurgery Executives' Resource Value & Education Society (NERVES, *www.nervesadmin.com*) and the Physician Office Managers Association of America (*http://pomaa.net*), to name just a few.

Talking to other professionals, your peers, is also a good idea. It's time to pick brains and not be shy about asking the tough questions, like how many patients you can expect each day and how much income you can expect per patient. Those estimates will have a significant effect on the number of people you need to hire, which will dramatically affect your proposed budget.

Budget will be addressed more closely in Essential # 5.

MANAGEMENT

Management is also part of your business plan, because it determines how many people you hire and what types of skills and job descriptions they have. Here are some important questions to ask yourself:

- Will you have an office manager or administrator?
- Will you act as your own office manager until your practice gets rolling?
- Will you have nurses? How many?
- Will you have physician assistants or nurse practitioners? How many?
- Will any of your staff be part-time or full-time?

The answer to these questions will build your practice's management structure, which will affect your budget. Those needs may change—will most assuredly change—as your practice gets going, but it's a place to start when it comes to visiting your friendly neighborhood loan officer with your hand out.

Although this can seem overwhelmingly complicated, bank loan officers are fairly experienced in dealing with physicians and other business people. Coming prepared will make them—and you—far happier. Come with a roadmap and your trip will be more likely to go smoothly.

"Typically, when you're budgeting for a start-up, you need about
6 months of working capital for both your business and personal budget."

HAT IN HAND

If you already have a relationship with a hospital, then it's obvious that you will want to keep privileges at that facility. First, for performing surgery, should that be necessary. Second, less obvious, are the marketing aspects. You will receive referrals from the primary care physicians at the hospital, which can run throughout numerous areas of the institution.

So, how many hospitals?

Geography plays a role. In a rural area, there may only be 1 hospital in the area and that may be enough. In an urban setting, it may have more to do with your particular area of expertise and the hospital's focus.

You typically need to apply through the specific department of your specialty or through human resources, or, more often, the medical staff office. In some cases, if the institution is particularly prestigious or there is a lot of competition for your specialty, you may find yourself having to "apply to apply." That is, before the institution will allow you to even apply for privileges, they will have to decide whether you're eligible to apply. This can depend on what boards certifications you have, where your residency was performed, etc.

Once you've completed the application and it is reviewed by the staff, you will typically be called in for an interview. Often, your application will then go to yet another committee, dubbed the Credentials and Qualifications Committee, then on to the Medical Executive Committee and, finally, to the Board of Directors. Hopefully, you will receive a stamp of approval from each committee. The entire process generally takes 3–4 months and sometimes as long as 6 months.

It is fairly common for your arrangement with the hospital to require your bringing in a certain number of patients per year; for example, 6 patients per year is typical, although some institutions require 12. In addition, you will be required to attend a certain number of meetings annually.

How many hospitals you're affiliated with is up to you, but some hospitals frown on competition and may place limits on how many competitors you can send patients to.

Also, in that the hospitals will be placing minimum patient referrals on your practice, it's worthwhile to think conservatively about just how many patients you're going to be sending to the hospital.

> *"It is fairly common for your arrangement with the hospital to require your bringing in a certain number of patients per year; for example, 6 patients per year is typical, although some institutions require 12."*

BEGGERS CAN'T BE CHOOSERS

You will also need to affiliate yourself with a number of third-party payers. Most of these carriers have an application fee of $200 or $250, so, although you may want, in the long run, to bring on as many carriers as possible, there may initially be financial limitations. Our recommendation is, however, to apply to as many as possible, because some of them will have 1- and 2-year waiting lists.

The biggest problem with having 30 third-party payers is that each will have different rules, requirements and reimbursements, which puts a strain on your administrative duties. Also, the more complicated the administrative duties, the more likely mistakes will happen.

There are, of course, a number of companies you will want to be aligned with: Medicare and Blue Cross, for instance.

Generally speaking, you will want the major government programs and the largest commercial carriers; then there will typically be more HMOs and PPOs based on your location.

Although there's no given number of third-party payers to be affiliated with, we believe it's best not to have any single payer account for more than 25% of your business. If, for some reason, you decide not to provide services to that carrier, it will have a significant impact on your business; vice versa, if there's something that would prevent you from working with that carrier, you'll be in trouble.

> *"Although there's no given number of third-party payers to be affiliated with, we believe it's best not to have any single payer account for more than 25% of your business."*

You will quickly find that not all third-party payers are created equal. When you're starting out, you may not be able to do much about that. After you've been in business a few years, you will probably want to evaluate your relationship with your payers. The best focus under the current health care economic landscape is to strive for the most efficient and effective patient volume, not necessarily the maximum patient volume.

Evaluate your variable expenses per patient and determine if a particular carrier reimburses at a level that sustains that level of expense. We recommend evaluating this at least annually. Many practices, as they mature, discover they are losing money on a significant percentage of their patients—10%, 15%, sometimes even 20%—and aren't even aware of it, because the third-party payer contracts have been modified so many times and additional fees charged that the dynamics have changed for the worse.

In other words, with some insurers, you may be losing money on those patients.

> **Action Step:** Create a business plan as discussed in this chapter, focusing on areas of your practice that need growth or improvement. Be specific, and have action plans and plans for regular monitoring.

Choosing Your Corporate Structure

The accountant's alphabet soup:
C-Corp, S-Corp, LLC, PC.

This section comes with a disclaimer. We are not attorneys. Before incorporating, consult an expert.

That said, there are 3 reasons to incorporate: 1, asset protection; 2, tax considerations; 3, succession planning.

Although your options may vary from state to state, and each provides different types of coverage in terms of options, there are generally 3 types of corporate entities:

1. Sole proprietorships
2. Limited liability companies (LLCs)
3. Business corporations

The professional corporation (PC) is a common operating structure for physicians. The primary difference between a sole proprietorship and a PC is that, if you are sued, a lawsuit can jeopardize your personal assets in a sole proprietorship; a PC limits nonmalpractice liability to just the corporation's assets.

For instance, if a patient falls on your sidewalk and sues you, the lawsuit is limited to only corporate assets. Another example is if you have a practice partner who is sued for malpractice for a patient you have not treated; only your partner and the corporation are liable. You are not.

> *"The professional corporation (PC) is a common operating structure for physicians. The primary difference between a sole proprietorship and a PC is that, if you are sued, a lawsuit can jeopardize your personal assets in a sole proprietorship; a PC limits nonmalpractice liability to just the corporation's assets."*

The limited liability company (LLC) is also quite common as a professional entity. In addition, there is something called a "limited liability partnership" or LLP. It's a partnership that provides liability protection similar to an LLC or PC. This category is becoming increasingly popular with physicians.

The advantage of an LLC is that the taxation is much simpler than a regular corporation, such as a PC, and simpler still than an S corporation.

Furthermore, some states do not allow physicians to use the business corporation structure. Oregon and Washington, are examples.

When discussing business corporations or PCs, there are subchapters S and C, usually referred to as an "S corp" or "C corp."

It is possible to set up a corporation for yourself using software. An example is *www. mycorporation.com*. *LegalZoom.com* also handles many business details online. However, although setting up a corporation is undoubtedly simpler than getting through medical school, there are nuances that are better handled by an expert. An example is, for instance, that if you set up an LLC, you'll need an operating agreement if your practice will have multiple practitioners in it.

Also, this is a definite case of screw-up-now-and-pay-later.

There are typically 3 questions you need to be able to answer before choosing a corporate structure.

- *How many people do you work with?* If you're a sole practitioner, you set it up that way. The question that quickly comes up though is, will you remain a sole practitioner? If you can envision someday bringing on a partner, it affects how you should set up your corporate structure.

- *What are your business goals?* If being a physician or a sole practitioner is the limit of your goals, that's fairly straightforward. If you envision that you might own a building and rent part of it, then your corporate structure may involve estate planning. If you can envision, for instance, owning buildings or multiple practices, or a laboratory or other business entities, these might need to be divided up because of either liability exposure or tax issues—-local, state and federal. These decisions affect your corporate structure.

- *Do you like business formalities?* Different corporate entities involve varying types of paperwork, officers and annual meetings. If you set up a more formal corporate entity, but then don't follow through with all the varying formalities, you may be undermining your liability protection. If you like doing that or at least don't mind doing it, fine; if you don't, recognize it early so your corporate structure won't become a headache.

And one final point: Corporations require a name. A good attorney or accountant can set up your corporate structure to minimize taxes and maximize liability protection. But what do you name your corporation?

The obvious choice is after yourself: "Johnny Appleseed, MD, PC." But it's so obvious, you might want to think of alternatives, should you decide to someday sell your practice. In that case, something like "Orion Doctors" or "Oakland County Physicians" may be more appropriate.

> **Action Step:** Speak to your accountant and discuss which corporate structure would be best for you based on your current needs and plans for future growth, both professionally and personally.

Developing A Budget

Budget for the first year, budget for every year.

A s mentioned earlier, your budget will essentially have 2 components: business and personal. However, there are 2 sides to the budget: cost and revenue.

To develop a cost budget, you need to have determined certain things about your practice. In a broad sense, they break down to 3 categories: space, equipment and staffing. You will need to know what type of practice you are running, how much space you will need and where it will be, what type of equipment you will need, whether you will rent or own (both equipment and your space), the types of staff you will require, how many, and how much you will pay them and what type of benefits you will offer them.

From that point, you need to determine what you will require for the first 6 months, what you will need by the end of the first year, and what you will need to be effective and efficient in operating your practice.

Once you have determined these components of your cost budget, you can develop a business plan that will look at a number of factors that will drive your budget: advertising, insurance, benefits, corporate and practice structure.

Now that you've started to develop the cost structure of your practice, you have to sit down and determine how much it will cost you to live. The components of that are straightforward: mortgage or rent, car payments, gas and insurance expenses, credit card debts and other loan payments, essentials such as food, utilities, etc.

For example, having worked out a cost budget for your practice, you have determined that it will take $15,000 a month to operate the practice. Having calculated your personal budget, you've determined that your personal cost budget is $6,000 per month. Combined, you need to generate $21,000 per month. This is the cost side of your budget.

You now turn to the revenue side of your budget. How much can you expect to be paid for each visit for each patient that comes through your door? This varies depending on your specialty. The Medical Group Management Association (*www.mgma.com*) has excellent benchmarking data on specialties as well as calculators to help determine how your budget and expenses compare to the national average. In addition, any professional organization related to your specialty will usually have benchmarking data available.

For the sake of simplicity, you've looked up your per patient revenue average through your professional organization and it is $100 per patient per visit. In order for you to meet your $21,000 monthly budget, you will need to have 210 patient visits per month.

From that point, you now know how many patients you need through your door and the average amount of income per patient you need to generate. Now you can create a somewhat circular equation to determine if you have enough money in your practice budget to make contacts and develop referral sources in order to generate 210 patients per month through advertising, marketing and communication.

> *"There are loose percentage benchmarks that you can expect to hit*
> *in your total budget, although it will vary from specialty to specialty.*
> *For instance, in podiatry, we generally expect 20%–25% of the budget*
> *to go toward salaries, wages and benefits; 5%–7% to go toward rent;*
> *2%–3% to go toward advertising; 8%–10% for medical supplies;*
> *and 3%–4% for office supplies."*

Other cost factors you will need to consider are repairs and maintenance, postage, contract management services, billing (in-house vs contracting outside), security, disposal of medical waste, telephone, cell phone expenses, Internet expenses, etc.

There are loose percentage benchmarks that you can expect to hit in your total budget, although it will vary from specialty to specialty. For instance, in podiatry, we generally expect 20%–25% of the budget to go toward salaries, wages and benefits; 5%–7% to go toward rent; 2%–3% to go toward advertising; 8%–10% for medical supplies; and 3%–4% for office supplies.

Again, those percentages will vary depending on your specialty and may shift somewhat, depending on the age and maturity of your practice as well as geographical location. Your professional organization or the MGMA will also have benchmarking data for your specialty.

Mike Crosby, president of Provider Resources, LLC (Brentwood, TN) assisted in the writing of this chapter. To contact, go to www.providerresources.com.

A FISTFUL OF DOLLARS

One of the toughest questions to answer: How much do you pay your staff?

First, you need to have a job description and job title, that way you have something to compare. Second, realize that you need to create a range, not just a specific number. If you hire an inexperienced person for the job, you want to be able to pay them more as they gain experience and mature as an employee. Obviously, if they stay with you long enough, they may max out that range, but if you don't set a range, you may price the employee out of the market and pay too much.

Pay ranges also vary from region to region. Several sources to investigate are:

1. Local medical organizations or societies in your city or state.
2. Local hospitals.
3. Colleagues in the area.
4. Temp agencies. Typically, temp agencies have higher pay rates because they don't offer benefits, but will provide a going rate for the position.

5. The Medical Group Management Association sells national data to its members. Their Web site is *www.mgma.com*.
6. Your state's employment commission.

Of course, when hiring someone, a useful question is: "What is your expected salary?" Another useful question: "What was your previous salary?"

If they have no training, you need to be up front that they'll start near the bottom and they will need to be trained. If they have experience, typically you'll meet their salary demands, unless they are unreasonable.

We suggest, either way, that you promise salary reviews at 3 months, 6 months and the 1-year anniversary. If your compensation was less than they expected, it's appropriate that within 3–6 months you will consider increasing their pay.

BALANCE AND BENEFITS

Deciding how much to pay your staff is only part of the equation and probably the easiest part. A more complicated issue is health benefits, vacation pay, paid time off and retirement packages. Again, you can fall back on your local standards as a benchmark. Talking with colleagues in the area will give you a good idea of what your local pay scales are like.

> *"For example, you might normally pay someone $18 an hour if they don't take benefits, but you pay them $14 an hour with benefits. That may be roughly equivalent, but it needs to be made very clear to the employee that the extra $4 is in lieu of benefits, so if they do ever decide they need medical benefits, they won't expect to continue to be paid $18 an hour plus the benefits."*

As of this writing—and we have no sense that this will change soon—medical benefits for employees are becoming increasingly expensive. More and more, employers are capping medical benefits at a specific value instead of, for instance, paying for medical benefits for an entire family, no matter how big it is.

It's important, if possible, to be flexible. Some people may take relatively low pay if they get health benefits for their family, because their spouse's employment may not offer health benefits. For example, you might normally pay someone $18 an hour if they don't take benefits, but you pay them $14 an hour with benefits. That may be roughly equivalent, but it needs to be made very clear to the employee that the extra $4 is in lieu of benefits, so if they do ever decide they need medical benefits, they won't expect to continue to be paid $18 an hour plus the benefits.

Many employers do not offer health benefits to part-time employees; some begin with generous benefits and some offer benefits as an alternative to increased salaries. The key issue is to make sure the job applicant is aware of the options before they take the job.

Some practice management consultants put together a spreadsheet for physicians to show potential employees' base salary, the costs of the benefits, plus the cost of vacation, sick time, etc, so they can see what the total compensation package is. We also encourage physicians to review total compensation with their employees on an annual basis, typically through a Compensation and Benefits Statement. This way, everybody's on the same page—also, they are made aware that in some cases salaries may be rising slowly, but the costs of benefits may be rising very quickly.

It's also important to know who your competitors are. A private medical practice usually cannot compete with a local hospital for salaries and benefits. However, a private medical practice can usually offer other compensations, such as flexible work hours, flexible start and stop times, flexible daily schedules and holidays off.

Some of what you decide will be based on your own practice's economics and on your own philosophy. Some of it, however, will be determined by your local economy and how fierce the competition is for good employees.

Action Step: Create an annual practice budget, including all key areas, and review it with your accountant. A good exercise to do while working on your budget is to look for areas for cost containment with a solid plan to reduce costs in those areas. Creativity is the key.

Hiring Your Staff

**Behind every successful doctor is an efficient staff.
How many people should you hire and what skills should they have?**

How many people should you hire? The answer is, as usual: it depends. First, however, ask yourself 4 questions:

1. How many physicians are there in the practice?
2. Do you plan to offer ancillary services?
3. How many locations do you have or plan to have?
4. Is the billing going to be performed in-house?

Having answered those 4 questions, you then need to consider what types of tasks you're expecting will be accomplished. For instance:

- Answering the phone(s)
- Making appointments
- Taking insurance information
- If you're billing in-house, you will need a manager or billing person
- Back office assistant
- Medical records-type activities

These are bare minimum nonmedical jobs in a typical doctor's office. There is also a technology component to your decision making: Will you have an answering machine or an answering service? Will you have an electronic appointment program, electronic billing systems, electronic medical records?

> *"If you're starting your practice, hiring a lot of people right from the get-go can also be cost-prohibitive. Many practice management consultants recommend beginning with an office manager and possibly 1 technician and a medical assistant or nurse. If you perform surgery in your practice, you may need more core staff. Typically, most consultants suggest 3½ staff per physician.*
> *"Another rule of thumb is you need 1½ front office staff for every 1 back office staff."*

If you do decide to lean heavily on digital medical records and other electronic services, keep in mind that the people you hire will either need to be thoroughly trained (as you yourself may need to be) or have experience with these types of technologies.

If you're starting your practice, hiring a lot of people right from the get-go can also be cost-prohibitive. Many practice management consultants recommend beginning with an office manager and possibly 1 technician and a medical assistant or nurse. If you perform surgery in your practice, you may need more core staff. Typically, most consultants suggest 3½ staff per physician.

Another rule of thumb is you need 1½ front office staff for every 1 back office staff.

Another way of determining number of staff involves looking at money. In this case, typical medical practices function best when their payroll ratio is 20%–22%. That is to say: Payroll and whatever health benefits or other benefits you intend to provide make up 20%–22% of the amount of collections annually. If you expect your practice to bring in $1,000,000 annually, then your payroll should be around $200,000–$220,000.

That is just for support staff and doesn't include your salary.

> *"Typical medical practices function best when their payroll ratio is 20%–22%. That is to say: Payroll and whatever health benefits or other benefits you intend to provide make up 20%–22% of the amount of collections annually. If you expect your practice to bring in $1,000,000 annually, then your payroll should be around $200,000–$220,000."*

Warning! When you're starting out, it's tempting to decide that, since you're not busy with patients, you'll skimp on staff and handle it yourself until you get busy; that you will answer the phones and do all your appointments, etc.

However, we feel strongly that when you're doing this you're cutting your own productivity. At this point in your practice's history, you would be much better off out shaking hands with other physicians who might send you referrals and performing various marketing activities to increase your patient load rather than answering your phones.

And finally, many physicians decide that early on in their practice they will handle the medical aspects of the practice and have their spouse (if their spouse is not also a physician) handle the office. There have certainly been many examples of this working well.

Our advice? In a group practice, never ever have a spouse running the office. Who's going to fire her/him if things don't work out? It just complicates matters entirely too much.

If you're just starting out and it's a solo practice, there are a lot of positives: 1, your spouse will work cheap (usually) if need be; 2, they're typically highly motivated to see the practice to do well.

On the negative side, be wary of any tensions. Other staff members may resent the spouse's presence and may not be completely candid when discussing problems that are occurring in the practice when the spouse is present.

This is also keeping in mind, of course, that your spouse may not actually be qualified for the job.

Recommendations if you do hire a spouse?

- Keep work at work and home life at home.
- Let your other employees know what's going on. If your spouse runs the office, will it be permanent? Do they have a chance for promotion if s/he's there?
- Put your spouse's duties in writing, just as you would with any other employee.
- Treat your spouse the same way you treat the rest of your staff.

What skills should you look for in an employee?

Although this might seem obvious, before you can decide what traits to look for, you need a job description. You may think, "Oh, I need a medical receptionist," without actually thinking about what skills that might entail. Yes, you might very well want a jack-of-all-trades that you can assign anything and everything to, but that rarely works in the real world. Better to know exactly what the job description is, so you can look for those skills.

This gets into a philosophical area, but we think it's an important one: hire for personality.

Yes, by all means look at resumes and conduct interviews about their abilities. Keep in mind, of course, that if you're just starting out, the most experienced employees also cost the most. So in that respect, you're better off looking for someone willing to learn.

It is our contention, however, that when you hire someone who has a can-do attitude, you can train them in most job responsibilities, they're easier to work with and will grow along with your practice.

During the interview, many interviewers find that doing a little role-playing can tell you more about an applicant's behavior then just answering questions. An example: Pretend to be an irate patient on the phone to see how the applicant responds to a cranky SOB that won't hang up.

Technologically savvy or at least technologically open-minded. This doesn't come up too often in discussions, but anyone who's tried to train an employee who has no computer experience and, furthermore, *doesn't want to have anything to do with computers* will understand when we suggest that someone who's open-minded about technology is a real plus in a medical office.

We also suggest that during an interview you work from a worksheet or checklist of specific questions and scenarios you wish to cover. This allows you to stay on track during the interview without posing any discriminatory questions or wandering off on tangents. More importantly, it makes your interviews more consistent so you can fairly and rationally evaluate each candidate.

The old adage is: Hire for attitude, train for success.

Still, don't overlook experience. Some people "give good interview" but won't necessarily work out in the office.

Some points are worth repeating. It's rare that 1 employee will be able to do all jobs. What you, as an employer, need to do is decide which skills a job requires and determine if a potential employee has those skills or can be trained in those tasks.

Aside from, say, being able to type or having memorized the entire ICD-10 catalogue (which would be both useful and impressive, no matter how unlikely), there are certain skills that are useful in an employee:

- Ability and willingness to take direction
- Ability to work with others
- Speed and mental processing
- Analytical skills

Questions that can lead you during the job interview to an evaluation of the potential employee's skills are:

- How do you determine your priorities?
- How do you plan your day? Week?
- What special characteristics should I know about you?
- Why are you interviewing with us?
- Can you give an example of how you've shown initiative and willingness to work?
- If you were doing the hiring, what would you be looking for?
- What was your former job's biggest challenge?
- How many levels of management did you interact with on your previous position?
- What kind of work interests you most?
- Describe your ideal job.
- How do you choose between 2 competing priorities?
- What is the toughest communication problem you have faced?
- Has there ever been a case where you have needed to follow up a verbal communication with a written communication?
- Describe an incident in a previous workplace where someone lost his or her temper with you.
- Have you ever worked in a place where it seemed to be just 1 crisis after another? How did you handle it? How did you feel?
- Define cooperation.
- What qualities should a successful manager possess?
- How have previous managers gotten the best out of you?
- Describe the best manager you've ever had. Describe the toughest manager you've ever had.
- For what have you been most frequently criticized?

Getting the best out of a new hire without tripping over illegal questions.

Having given you a number of questions you should ask or consider asking in an interview, and suggested role-playing as a method for getting a sense of how a potential employee may behave, we want to address the often sticky topic of what you can't ask in a job interview.

First, if you have some doubt as to the legality of a particular question, consult with an attorney familiar with labor laws. Due to the myriad laws covering this subject, it can be a minefield.

SUBJECT	ILLEGAL QUESTIONS	SUGGESTED ALTERNATIVES
National Origin/ Citizenship	Are you a US citizen? Where were you/parents born?	Are you authorized to work in the US? What languages do you read, speak or write fluently? (This question is appropriate if language ability is relevant to performance of the job).
Age	How old are you? When did you graduate from college? What is your birthday?	Are you over the age of 18? Tell me about your education.
Marital/Family Status	What's your marital status? Who do you live with? Do you plan to have a family? When? How many children do have? What are your child care arrangements?	Would you be willing to relocate? We have multiple offices and travel is an important part of the job. Would you be willing to travel as needed by the job? (Appropriate if all applicants are asked the same question.) This job sometimes requires overtime. Are you able and willing to work overtime as necessary? (Again, appropriate if all applicants are asked it.)
Affiliations	What clubs or social organizations do you belong to?	Do you belong to any professional or trade groups or other organizations that you consider relevant to your ability to perform this job?
Personal	How tall are you? How much do you weigh?	Are you able to lift a 50-pound weight and carry it 100 yards? (Only if that skill is part of the job. Questions about height and weight are not acceptable unless minimum standards are essential to the safe performance of the job.)
Disabilities	Do you have any disabilities? Have you had any recent or past illnesses or operations? What was the date of your last physical exam? How's your family's health?	Are you able to perform the essential functions of this job with or without reasonable accommodations? (This question is appropriate if the interviewer thoroughly described the job.)
Arrest Record	Have you ever been arrested?	Have you ever been convicted of_____? (The crime should be reasonably related to the performance of the job in question.)

Action Step: Determine your optimum staffing in each area of your office—front office, clinical, back office and billing. Create an interview protocol and questions to use for future recruiting. Be as detailed as possible. Make a list of mistakes you have made in the past when interviewing.

Leadership Skills

How to manage your staff and keep your headaches to a minimum.

Character is the major trait of an effective leader. What decisions you make and how you make them filter down to your staff, and affects how your patients do and how they perceive you and your practice.

- Empower your staff, don't micromanage them. Provide clear and consistent feedback. Celebrate your staff's achievements publicly so everyone can see, and discipline their shortcomings quietly and in private. Criticize the behavior, not the individual.

- Listen to input from your staff and employees. They should be encouraged to provide input to your plans that will help achieve your practice's goals. Lead, don't dictate—be a leader, not a dictator. Manage from the bottom up—the people who have to implement your plans may have better ideas on how to implement them because they're the ones who have to do it.

- Be realistic. Employees are not machines and do not operate as consistently as machines. Everyone has a bad day.

- Be fiscally responsible. Know how your practice's finances work. Be on top of what's going on both medically and financially.

- Focus on the present *and* the future. Staff meetings are about creating a dialogue with your staff. Understand what's going on now and how it can affect future actions.

- Don't ask your staff to do things you would not be willing to do yourself. Pitch in on the miserable jobs if you have time—lead by example.

- Pay attention to communication styles—yours and your staff's. Not all people communicate the same way. Some people require repetition and follow-up; others feel that repetition is nagging and means you don't trust them to do the job. Some people require regular feedback on their performance (minute by minute, hour by hour) while others don't want any comment until they are completed. Being aware of the differences will make life easier and smoother for everyone involved.

- Become a proactive listener. Don't just hear . . . *listen!*

- Remember the Golden Rule and its corollary, the Bounce-Back Rule: Whatever you dish out . . . bounces back! (What goes around, comes around).

- Verbal communication is only about 40% of communication. Remember eye contact, body language, voice intonation, volume and inflection.

- And finally, be your staff's advocate and protector. Remember, great leaders don't just lead and create a direction; they create an umbrella of safety for the people they are leading. Many employees say they don't mind if their boss is demanding if they know he or she values them, recognizes that value and defends them to others. This places the leader in a different role than just "boss" or "employer" but reminds you that these people—their jobs, their welfare, and well-being and yes, even happiness, are your responsibility.

> *"Manage from the bottom up—the people who have to*
> *implement your plans may have better ideas on how to implement*
> *them because they're the ones who have to do it."*

WHO'S THE FIRST MATE?

By now you've hired your staff, you're seeing patients and things are progressing. You are the captain of your ship, so to speak, but you can't do everything. You're busy doing that thing that brings in money—being a doctor.

So, although you need to know what's going on in your office, you really need someone to depend on to monitor and oversee the day-to-day operations of your practice. In keeping with the ship metaphor, you're looking for a first mate (or executive officer).

Typically, this person is your office manager or administrator.

One of the first impulses of a boss is to promote people that are just like themselves. Sometimes this works. Sometimes it doesn't.

Often a doctor will promote the employee they like the most, who may not necessarily be the best person for the job.

Something that is often forgotten about our office managers—and our staff in general—is that they are *not* assistants or backroom staff. They are professionals and an extension of you.

So one of the key ingredients you should look for in an office manager is: professionalism.

Another: Willingness to learn. They will need to set an example for the rest of the staff, because a practice that doesn't grow and change with demands is likely to wither and die.

Don't hire a "yes man." This is a huge temptation, often subconscious, because, after all, you tend to like people that agree with you all the time. But, there is a difference between someone who constantly disagrees with you and has a negative attitude and someone who speaks their own mind and gives you their honest opinion. You definitely will benefit from someone who will tactfully let you know when they think you're not doing something right.

And perhaps most of all, look for someone who can handle the responsibility.

THOUGHTS ON PROFESSIONAL ORGANIZATIONS FOR STAFF

Just as it's important for you, the physician, to be a lifelong learner, take part in continuing education, read journals and attend conferences, it's important that your staff stay educated and informed on what's going on in the field as well. After all, every aspect of health care is undergoing change these days, some of it quite dramatic.

Nurses have a number of professional organizations they can and often do belong to. The Medical Group Management Association (*www.mgma.com*) is an organization that office managers and administrators might consider joining. It's a large organization, with 21,500 members, which indicates it has a lot of clout, but can also be a bit intimidating for new members. There are a number of state chapters that can provide more intimacy and 1-on-1 interactions.

Another reasonable complaint about MGMA is the cost, which at this time is $365 per year with a one-time $95 application fee. That's pretty steep for an office manager or administrator, so if you as a physician feel it's important for some members of your staff to be members, you should offer to pay either some or all of the yearly fees.

Other associations exist as well, such as the Physician Office Managers Association of America (*www.pomaa.net*).

There are also a number of educational opportunities for staff, whether it's classes in coding, billing, office management, or computer technology or conferences and seminars that would be valuable for them to attend. Encouraging your staff to participate in these opportunities can emphasize that you feel they are professionals and part of their professional responsibility is to continue to educate themselves in their field.

> **Action Step:** List personality traits you possess that will make you a good leader and write your plans for the next 12 months, which should be reviewed on a regular basis. Ask everyone in your office to anonymously write what they feel your strengths and weaknesses are as a leader (and be sure to have tissues in hand!).

Marketing Your Practice, Part I

Practical steps to getting the patient in the door.

Much of your early business will come through referrals. In order to get referrals, you're going to need to go out into your community and meet physicians at the local hospitals and other practices. It's also a two-way street, because you will be meeting people you can refer to in the future as well.

In the current health care environment, primary care physicians serve as gatekeepers for all the specialty areas. That means, ultimately, if you are not a primary care physician, when you spend time developing a marketing plan, some of that plan will be focused on primary care physicians. (Yes, primary care physicians, you now have a bull's-eye painted on your back).

Typically, aside from the "Yeah, I know her, she's a great doc" type of referral, a primary care physician or any other referrer will be considering 3 things when deciding upon a referral: 1. The relationship between the referring physician and the specialist; 2. The timeliness of feedback regarding the patients' visits; 3. The competence of the specialist.

> *"In the current health care environment, primary care physicians serve as gatekeepers for all the specialty areas."*

Bottom line: You need to be considered user-friendly and cost-effective.

PLAN A: SHORT VISITS

1. Have your staff contact the office managers of primary care physician and specialists in your area. Have them ask for a short appointment lasting 5–10 minutes during lunch for a formal introduction or an informal hello.

2. When you go to the appointment, despite the admonition to "Beware of Greeks bearing gifts," bring a gift of some sort: desserts, cookies, a pie. Food often works well in this situation because you're involving the staff as well as the physician.

3. Ask if you can leave business cards. Also, many doctors note that leaving a pad of referral forms that the referring physician can give to patients works well. The form should include your practice's address, phone number, Web site and a map, as well as space for the patient's name, referring physician and diagnosis. Some referral forms include a checklist of the most common conditions likely referred for.

4. Follow up with a handwritten thank-you, either by you or on your behalf.

PLAN B: LUNCH AND LEARN

A "Lunch and Learn" is where you or, even better, a knowledgeable staffer, present mini-talks during lunch (which you may provide) to the referring physician's staff on what it is you do. Although this works well for physicians, in our experience, if you have a knowledgeable and articulate staffer, the referring physician's staff relate better.

1. Have the staffer contact the manager of the physician's office. He or she offers to bring lunch to the office staff to eat while listening to a short presentation.
2. The staffer, after giving a talk about, for example, a specific medical condition that they commonly treat, supplies the office staff with a professional packet. The packet should include a laminated list of contracted insurance plans, physician ID numbers, a pad of referral forms and any brochures concerning your specialty. You can also include Rolodex cards with your contact information.
3. Keep these "Lunch and Learn" visits between 30–45 minutes long.
4. The presenter can act as a contact person between the referral staff and yourself, and should leave a business card that indicates this.
5. Follow up with a handwritten thank-you, either by you or on your behalf.

PLAN C: HOLIDAY GIFTS

1. Food is always a good holiday gift, particularly one that can be shared by the entire staff.
2. T-shirts that someone might wear, but that also, in small print, includes the name of your practice.
3. For many gifts, have a member of your staff deliver the holiday basket in person so more introductions can be made.

PLAN D: EXPANSION

Whenever you add a physician, partner or additional ancillary service, send out announcements and a letter of introduction.

PLAN E: TRACKING THE COMPETITION

Pay attention to new physicians and practitioners in your area. Welcome them to the community and introduce yourself, letting them know about your own office protocols. Tell them you'd like to meet them in their office or for lunch. Offer an in-service lunch for their office.

PLAN F: CONTINUITY

Maintain the rapport. This is not a one-shot deal, nor is it a crass and commercial form of networking—referring physicians aren't just competition, but your peers and professional community. Stay in touch. Organize lunch dates and meetings. And above all, communicate with the referring physicians about their patients' treatment! This is the single most important part of the relationship. Provide top-level care for their patients and they'll continue to refer them to you.

Action Step: See Essential #9.

Marketing Your Practice, Part II

Internal and external marketing and tracking your efforts.

CREATING A BUDGET, LAUNCHING A CAMPAIGN AND FINDING YOUR FOCUS

D o armies go into war without a plan? No. When McDonald's rolls out a new product, do they just offer it up to their various restaurants and hope people will notice it on the menu between the Quarter Pounders and the Filet-O-Fish? No. So, what you need is a plan. In fact, you need a campaign for marketing your practice and bringing patients into your office. Although marketing never ends, it's better to decide first what it is you're trying to achieve, and then put into place certain actions and strategies that will help you achieve that goal. In our experience, many physicians don't organize their marketing campaign or think about what they're trying to accomplish. They are essentially shooting arrows without a target in front of them.

> *"Many physicians don't organize their marketing campaign or think about what they're trying to accomplish. They are essentially shooting arrows without a target in front of them."*

If you go back to Essential #1, we discussed what type of practice you want, what your mission statement is, how you've defined your practice. In the process of defining yourself and your practice, you should have answered questions like:
- Where do your patients come from?
- Where do your patients live?
- Who referred your patients to you?

Knowing now what type of practice you want helps create a "brand" for your practice and helps shape your marketing campaign. For example, if you're aiming at a geriatric or diabetic patient population, ads in your local college newspaper may be a waste of time. It seems obvious, but you'd be surprised at how often this sort of thing is overlooked.

Potential marketing avenues are:
- The Yellow Pages
- Web site
- Local and/or regional newspaper advertisements
- Direct mailings
- Lunches and talks with potential referring physicians

- Lunches and talks with local organizations such as the Kiwanis, Rotary Club, Chamber of Commerce
- Radio and TV advertisements
- Writing local newspaper columns
- Nursing home visits
- Event presentations/booths
- Open houses
- Referrals

These all fall into the category of external marketing (ie, marketing outside your practice). Internal marketing, on the other hand, refers to having brochures in your office, newsletters and how you treat your patients—suggest to them that if they're happy with your care, they should recommend you to a friend or relative.

It's important to evaluate your cost-vs-benefit ratio for each avenue. At one time, every doctor had to have a Yellow Pages ad, even though they're very expensive. However, in today's current climate, a Web site is required and a full-page Yellow Pages listing might be questionable, although a regular listing is probably still a good idea. Radio and TV costs and reach will vary a great deal depending on what market you're in—a large, urban market will have a huge reach, but you'll pay accordingly. A smaller, rural or suburban market may cost quite a bit less—even a TV ad through a local cable TV supplier—but will reach fewer people, although it may, as a result, be more targeted than a radio or TV ad in a large, urban market.

> *"A general rule of thumb is 10% of your projected revenues should be set aside from marketing."*

Of course, all of these decisions will be constrained by your marketing budget. And yes, when you created your budget, you needed to set aside money for marketing efforts. Although how much of your budget should go to marketing varies from consultant to consultant, a general rule of thumb is 10% of your projected revenues should be set aside for marketing.

And don't forget, as mentioned in Essential #8, getting out and meeting people—doctors, nursing homes, giving talks at local organizations, etc—is relatively inexpensive, although it can be time consuming.

But perhaps the most important thing to remember about marketing is that you really need more than 1 type of marketing format. A Web site alone won't do it, a Yellow Pages ad alone won't do it, direct mail alone won't do it, etc. It's helpful to think of your marketing campaign as a pie and, in order for it to be effective, you have to have as many different pieces of that pie in use as possible.

STRATEGIES FOR INTERNAL MARKETING

The previous section dealt primarily with external marketing/how to get patients into your office. In a new practice, you don't have much choice. But as patients start coming into your office, internal marketing can be a powerful tool.

Internal marketing, unlike external marketing, tends to be less about media—print, such as newspapers and flyers, or electronic, such as radio, TV and Internet—and more about processes that you can put into place. In other words, what types of behaviors do you and/or your staff have that become part of a marketing strategy?

Here are 10 ways you can internally market your practice.

1. Improve your communication skills. In other words, personal charisma—be a physician that patients like.
2. Interact both professionally and socially with primary care physicians who will then be glad to refer patients your way.
3. Make timely follow-up telephone calls to patients.
4. Get your reports back to your referring physicians in a timely fashion.
5. Have a brochure and business cards available in your office that indicate your areas of expertise and the conditions you treat.
6. Have brochures and other literature available for various diagnoses that can be given to the patient.
7. Be available—to patients and to referring physicians.
8. As simple as this seems, when patients calling your office are put on hold, make sure to have a cheerful, professional message and some sort of recording for them to listen to.
9. Make sure your office is an attractive place to visit—cheerful and bright.
10. When you have a satisfied patient, ask them to refer you to a friend or relative.

Internal marketing has a far stronger cost-vs-benefit ratio than external marketing and results in highly motivated, loyal patients.

Additional, but simple ideas of internal marketing are:

- Sending patients birthday cards and holiday greeting cards.
- Recontacting via phone calls, cards or letters. Just because a patient has been treated and released, doesn't mean that 6 months later you can't have a staffer give them a phone call and ask them how they're doing. This sort of courtesy and thoughtfulness can lead to return visits. A simple "How are you doing?" followed by a short, friendly conversation is sufficient, no sales pitch needed.
- Let patients know who you are. Have a book of you and your staff's accomplishments, awards and accolades. Frame newspaper articles about you and hang them on your office wall, including photographs of yourself giving talks or presentations at regional and national meetings.

- Don't forget good lighting in your office and even fresh flowers (unless you're an allergist, in which case, that might not be a good idea).
- Can you make your patients' lives easier? Do you have an on-site pharmacy or offer commonly sold medical items in your office, saving your patients a trip to the pharmacy or drug store? These services not only increase your bottom line, they save your patients time.
- Listen. That's part of being a good doctor, right? Listen to your patients and they will listen to you. Listen to your employees and you'll be a better boss. This is a skill worth cultivating.
- Be efficient. Don't make patients wait longer than 5–7 minutes in the reception room. Prepare for your day by going through your patients' charts and do as much standard prep, such as having pre-cut or ready-made padding done, ahead of time as possible—it saves time for everybody.

EVALUATING YOUR MARKETING EFFORTS

Keep it or scrap it? Ways to determine which marketing efforts work.

Although the expression has been attributed to several different people, including John Wanamaker (a 19th-century department store mogul), Henry Ford and JC Penney, there's a lot of truth to it: Half of every dollar spent on advertising and marketing is wasted, but since we don't know which half, we go ahead and spend the full dollar anyway.

One of the most frustrating things about marketing is many physicians create marketing campaigns and don't bother to see what works and what doesn't. Yet almost everything is trackable. We offer 7 methods for tracking your marketing efforts.

#1. Ask your patients how they got there.

Makes sense, right? Go to the source. When a new patient calls or walks in your door, you or your staff needs to simply ask, "So, how did you hear about us?" In fact, this is such an important question, we feel that it should be part of a drop-down menu on your practice management software that prompts you to ask the question.

But this isn't limited to just your staff, who should ask whenever a patient calls for an appointment. It needs to be an integral part of your practice's intake process.

#2. Take note!

In other words, having asked the patient for information, you now need to write it down somewhere, preferably included in your practice management software. For instance, if Mariah Jones refers Sandy Smyth, that referral needs to be placed under Mariah Jones' name. It's a good idea to not only note who referred whom, but how much money the referring patient spent in your practice. A quarterly review of this information might show you trends: maybe Mariah Jones is a regular referrer and has given you 5 new patients who brought in $15,000 of work. If so, you might want to help her with her balance or offer her some products as a HIPAA-compliant way of thanking her for all she's done for your practice.

One medical practice in Fort Collins, Colorado tracks all marketing efforts at the front desk. At the desk is a 4-column list that indicates every advertisement the physician uses, whether it's in the local newspaper, in a business journal or on the Internet. Once the question is asked, the response is checked off, then they look for more granularity to the data, for instance, asking which Yellow Pages ad it was or what newspaper. The physician and his staff then have a lunch meeting once a week, and they present all the statistics from the data so they can get a sense of what's working and what isn't and where to place their advertisements. This time and effort has really paid off financially.

> *"It's a good idea to not only note who referred whom,*
> *but how much money the referring patient spent in your practice.*
> *A quarterly review of this information might show you trends:*
> *maybe Mariah Jones is a regular referrer and has given you*
> *5 new patients who brought in $15,000 of work."*

#3. Code your materials.

Every time you have an advertisement, whether it's a flyer at a health fair, a newspaper ad, a Web site, Yellow Pages ad, brochure or even a letter to another physician, you should place a code of some sort on that document. It can be as simple as a #14 in the bottom left corner. This way, when someone calls in and you ask them how they found out about you, you or your staff can ask them to check the number code and you'll know exactly which media they're referring to.

#4. Create an incentive.

One way to create some urgency to your advertising is to include an incentive with it. This can be something like suggesting that if the patient mentions a particular flyer, or brings it into the office with them, they will receive something. For example, a $5 gas card or something similar.

#5. E-newsletters.

Using services like Constant Contact or Vertical Response, many physicians send e-newsletters to their patients. This inexpensive marketing technique can keep your practice on patients' radars. Keep them short and informative, and include plenty of information and photographs. Physicians who do this report strong recall responses.

#6. Analyze your Yellow Pages' return on investment.

The Yellow Pages used to be a rite of passage for all businesses. However, ads could cost up to $40,000 a year. The Internet has largely supplanted this big yellow dinosaur. So, if you are using the Yellow Pages, it would be a good idea to analyze how many patients you're getting in by it and whether it's paying for itself. Also, if your practice has been in existence for a while, when patients tell you they saw your ad in the Yellow Pages, ask them what page the ad was on. Some physicians have discovered that patients aren't necessarily using current Yellow Pages to find you.

#7. Analyze your Internet presence.

In the wider world of advertising and marketing, the Internet has caused a revolution, not only in terms of costs, but in terms of analysis. Search engines and Web site traffic analysis have allowed for targeted advertising and the creation of a tremendous amount of useful data about who's viewing your Web site and how—are they surfing in, finding you via search engines like Google or something smaller and local, or through your insurance company Web site links. By finding out this information, you can focus more of your marketing energies on what works and waste less time, money and energy on marketing black holes.

You should take tracking 1 step further, from merely tracking effectiveness to tracking return on investment. The 80/20 rule is a classic in many areas, and applies to marketing as well—80% of your business probably comes from about 20% of your patients, and 80% of your business comes from 20% of your marketing. The key is to figure out which 20%.

Looking at your patients and how much revenue they bring into your practice, then connecting those patients to referrals, marketing sources and revenue, you begin to have a sense of the financial value of a new patient. As podiatrists, we value a new patient at a minimum of $1,500. Over a 2-year period, an obstetrician may see $5,220 per household from a single patient, or only $760 per patient—depending, somewhat, on whether the patient is pregnant. The Internet Dental Directory indicates the average value of a new patient for a dentist is initially $3,000–$3,500, and about 10% of those patients have a 2-year worth of $15,000–$45,000. That may sound high initially, but if you take into consideration not just the services that patient will receive, but the potential referrals from that patient, it could go much higher. Much of it depends on the types of patients, but you can probably expect a typical satisfied patient to provide 2 referrals.

Ultimately it falls to 2 questions: How many patients did your marketing efforts bring in? And, how will you know if you don't track your marketing efforts?

> **Action Step:** Along with key team members, create your marketing budget and plan, focusing on both patient retention and development. What are your chief weaknesses in internal and external marketing? List 3 ways to improve them.

ESSENTIAL #10:

Writing Your Office Manual

What you need to know about your responsibilities as an employer.

The time to write your office manual is before you hire people, not after. Every employee should receive a copy of the office manual when they are hired and be required to read it and sign off that they've read and understood it. That agreement then needs to be included in their personnel file. Also, whenever your office manual is updated or modified, employees must read and sign off on the updates and their agreement should also be included in their personnel file.

An office manual takes all of your rules and policies—and even what might be called "work culture"—and puts it in writing. This puts everybody on the same page. Without having procedures in writing, employees may make assumptions about what is correct, whether about appropriate attire, how to make time-off requests, or appropriate Internet and phone usage, for example.

At its most basic, the manual should contain:
1. General information.
2. Explanations of benefits.
3. Safety procedures.
4. Policies and procedures.
5. Resignation and termination procedures.

There is no requirement as to length. Some physicians and their employees find that an office manual that is too long can be rather intimidating or overwhelming. Many find 30–40 pages about right; others choose to create 2 manuals, one that has employee and liabilities policies in it, and another for procedural information.

GENERAL INFORMATION

This section should contain information about the physician, the practice and include the practice's mission statement. It will also spell out the expectations of the employee for each job, describe the various employment levels in the practice, and whatever rules and regulations that exist.

Benefits

Your manual should describe the available benefits packages and include your practice's policies related to holidays, paid time off, absenteeism, insurance, retirement, maternity or family leave. You should plan to perform annual or semi-annual personnel evaluations, and your policy and approach to that should be described in the manual.

Safety Procedures

Your employee manual should include procedures and protocols for dealing with emergencies, whether related to patients, fire, tornado, etc. It should address accidents, injuries and OSHA compliance.

Policies and Procedures

This section should address more general office policies, including dress codes, telephone and Internet usage, lunch hours, breaks, attendance, parking, as well as policies related to smoking, drug use, alcohol abuse or other substance abuse. It can also include office hours, sick days, wages, overtime, bonus incentives, maternity and bereavement leaves, retirement plans, vacations and holidays, cross training, staff meetings, etc.

Resignation and Termination Procedures

How and why you fire someone can leave you and your practice open to litigation. Having a written policy in place that the employee has agreed to is not just good business, but could eliminate headaches in the future.

> *"If you have an office manual stating what the procedures are*
> *for an incident and you then terminated that person and didn't follow*
> *the procedures in the office manual, your defense in a wrongful*
> *termination suit or harassment lawsuit becomes largely nonexistent.*
> *So, it's not enough to just have an office manual, you have to follow*
> *what it says you're to do in various situations."*

There are a number of reasons besides good business practices to have an office manual. First, a great many harassment lawsuits are based on a practice's or business's lack of an office manual. Typically, this falls under the category of: if the employee claims to have been harassed, they were unaware of who to go to for a complaint. However, this can work against you as well; if you have an office manual stating what the procedures are for an incident and you then terminated that person and didn't follow the procedures in the office manual, your defense in a wrongful termination suit or harassment lawsuit becomes largely nonexistent. So, it's not enough to just have an office manual, you have to follow what it says you're to do in various situations.

Second, a number of states require a small business to have an office manual.

Third, many physicians find that having a good office manual results in less complaining from staff about the way things are done because what is expected is clearly stated in writing. People are just plain less likely to buck the system and do their own thing when you have the rules down on paper. Decision making becomes easier, simply because the rationale is already in print for tough decisions.

In addition to a section on policies and procedures, your office manual can include a section that covers day-to-day operations. This can range from information on how to file an insurance claim to how to chart a patient, even material on telephone procedures. It can also be broken up into front office and back office procedures. These can be particularly helpful when cross-training staff or for staff to lean on when filling in for other employees.

Also, a confidentiality protocol in compliance with HIPAA laws should be in place.

It's not necessary that you start from scratch when developing your manual. There are several software packages, including Office Policy Manual by WriteExpress, that can help you design an office manual for a fairly small amount of money. The American Academy of Family Physicians (AAFP) also offers an *Operational Procedures for the Physician Practice*, a customizable CD-ROM that will help you create an operational procedures manual tailored to your own practice. (*http://www.aafp.org/online/en/home/practicemgt/special topics/operational-procedures.html*). Many management consultants sell templates as well.

Start small, section by section. We also recommend that, when your manual is finished, you have it reviewed by an attorney that specializes in labor and employment issues. Although an office manual is designed to make sure everyone knows what your practice's rules and procedures are, in many ways it is a legal document that can protect your practice. You don't want to have things written in such a way as to cause you problems.

Your office manual should also be reviewed each year, not just by you, but by your staff and office manager. Ask for feedback. You might find some policies cause problems instead of solving them, or that they have become outdated. It's also useful to have an attorney review your manual yearly to make sure it's current with state and federal laws.

Action Step: Craft (or update) your office manual. Ask 1 or 2 physicians in your area if you can review their office manuals for ideas on how to improve yours.

ESSENTIAL #11:
Office Dynamics: The "EFF" Words

Being EFFicient and EFFective with minimum EFFort—
developing systems for your practice.

How you operate your practice—from who accompanies you in to see the patient to how the phones are answered and how patients are led to the consulting rooms—tends to evolve. The problem is that it may not evolve in an effective, efficient manner. This can lead to a we've-always-done-it-that-way attitude that can be difficult to change.

It's far better to have *directed evolution*—to think about how you do things, how you want to do things, and set into place systems that you and your staff can use as a roadmap to accomplishing your practice's goals.

1. *Plan Ahead.* Not just for how you want to set things up, but for how you want your day to run. Many physicians arrive to work an hour or so early to look over the day's schedule and develop a game plan. How much time should you spend with each patient? Barring surprises—and there are always surprises—some patients may only require 5 or 10 minutes, while others will require 30. Decisions regarding organizing appointments are affected by what the patient is coming in for, while other times it's merely the patient's personality—Mrs. Johnston sure does love to talk.

   If there are x-rays to look at, now may be the time to do it, not 30 seconds before you enter the examining room. A lot will depend on how you personally approach patient care, but setting a course through your day will help you stay on track.

2. *Communicate.* It's important that your staff understand what you want to achieve and how you think it should be done, but it's equally—perhaps even more so—important that you listen to your staff. By recording and analyzing your own activities and those of each of your staff members, everyone will begin to anticipate each other's needs in best servicing your patients.

   For instance, Hal found that if his staff thoroughly explained procedures to patients and addressed their concerns, he could provide more comprehensive care to a larger number of patients. The trick is to communicate with your staff while still respecting everybody's duties and responsibilities.

3. *Focus On The Patient.* What is your practice's primary goal? Hopefully, to meet and exceed patient expectations. The reason for a physician practice's existence is the care of patients. Anything that detracts from that goal should be evaluated with a cold, clear eye to see why it's being done that way. How does everybody's actions improve the overall care the patient is receiving?

"The reason for a physician practice's existence is the care of patients.
Anything that detracts from that goal should be evaluated with
a cold, clear eye to see why it's being done that way."

4. *Momentum Starts At The Top.* Although there's a lot to be said for listening to your staff and paying attention to their suggestions on how things should be done—after all, they are the ones who do it every day—you as the head of the practice set the tone and lead by example. Your staff follows your lead. If you're unorganized and distracted, they will tend to be as well. If you do things on the fly and improvise, they will too.

5. *Prioritize.* We heard this story at a management workshop. The speaker held up a vase and then filled it with large rocks. He asked the audience if it was full. They said it was, but he then poured small pebbles into it, which sifted down to the bottom of the vase. Asked if it was full yet, the audience indicated that yes, they thought so. The speaker then poured sand into the vase, which filled in the spaces between the pebbles. Full yet? The audience thought so, but the speaker then filled the vase with water.

   It's an obvious analogy for prioritizing. A physician's ability to create income is finite; there are limits to it. Many doctors respond to a need for increased revenue by extending their hours. Although that may be okay with limits, it's also a surefire way to hop on the gerbil wheel and exhaust yourself. Burnout both professionally and personally can result.

   What gives you the most satisfaction? What can only you do? (Hopefully, they're pretty much the same things). That's what you need to focus on. You should see patients, but there's no reason your staff can't do some of the basics, like patient intake, blood pressure, pulse, temperature, discussing future appointments or describing durable medical equipment, thus freeing you up to see other patients.

6. *Create Protocols.* One simple way to streamline your practice and become more effective and efficient is to create written protocols, or checklists of what needs to be done and said. A checklist of questions that ask things like:
   - *How long have you been suffering with this condition? Days/ Weeks/ Months/Longer*
   - *Is this condition affecting your ability to perform daily tasks? Yes / No*

   Of course, 1 form does not fit all. But having forms for your practice's most common diagnoses is a step toward making sure there is consistency in how you approach the work.

   Taking that 1 step further, do you provide ancillary services, like physical therapy, or have an on-site pharmacy? Do you dispense durable medical equipment? It's surprising how many physicians and their staffs offer these services, but fail to mention them to their patients. Reminding yourself to mention these on your SOPs will bring in surprising dividends in terms of efficiency and increased revenue.

Action Step: List 5-10 changes that you and your team can make immediately to enhance your efficiency. Be sure to take baby steps or little may change.

ESSENTIAL #12:

Motivating Your Staff

Inspiration, not perspiration, gets the most out of your employees.

Many studies of workplace motivation have found that money is not the primary motivating factor for most employees. Unfortunately, many practitioners and business owners in general have jumped on that concept as if it were the answer to prayers—*"Our staff will be satisfied with a pat on the back and a heartfelt thank you."*

No, not quite. Underpay, don't give out regular and reasonable bonuses, don't provide competitive salaries and benefits, and your practice will run into trouble soon enough as your office becomes a revolving door for staff looking for better jobs.

Nonetheless, in terms of motivation, factors vary. Some people, it's true, will only be motivated by money. For others it may be simple verbal positive reinforcement, for instance, telling them, "Great job!"

Some people like to use incentives for a job well done by providing a small reward, such as a gift card or flowers or monthly plaque. We're not opposed to any of those, although just be aware that this can backfire. Mark worked at a company whose boss decided to reward staffers who he thought had done something worth praising with a "Cracker Jack Award," which consisted of a small box of Cracker Jack. This rather quickly became a joke among the staffers, that in lieu of a year-end bonus or a competitive wage, they were given a 75-cent box of caramel popcorn and peanuts. Also, since the reasons for the "award" were fairly arbitrary, such as someone working 15 minutes late or solving a particularly knotty problem, it created a fair amount of resentment among the rest of the staffers. A common refrain was that one person got an award for something that everybody else routinely did. The success of this sort of thing may largely depend on the overall morale or the personalities of your staffers.

You also have to be careful that, if you're going to do this kind of thing on a regular basis, like once a month, the same person doesn't keep winning the "award" or receiving the "incentive."

Making this work involves knowing your staff well enough to know what they will respond to best. Financial incentives often are the most productive, but the amount required can be minimal (although Cracker Jack might be too minimal) if used synergistically and consistently with other nonfinancial rewards.

Financial rewards should be linked to hitting some sort of goal, and that goal should be agreed upon by both you and your staffer. In order to maximize the effectiveness of an incentive, it needs to be under the control of the staff member who will receive the bonus.

Examples:

#1. Staffer: Billing and collections
Goal: Set a predetermined collection goal.

#2. Staffer: Receptionist
Goal: Improve rate of collecting deductibles and copayments.

Above all, the incentive needs to be consistent, fair, ethical and in the best interest of the practice. Incentive programs that aren't can be much worse than never having one at all.

It is also very important that you, as a manager, provide the resources the staffer needs to achieve the desired outcome.

For a medical practice, we offer 6 examples of outcomes that can be linked to a financial incentive program.

1. An increase in gross monthly collections, the collection of overdue (aged) accounts or the net collection ratio.
2. An increase in the number of new scheduled patients.
3. An increase in in-office dispensing revenues.
4. Growth in the number of patient visits.
5. Well-received results of patient satisfaction surveys.
6. Satisfactory (or better) results on an annual employee review.

DETERMINING THE GOAL

A goal needs to be reached by studying your practice's history. Yes, that's tricky if you're a new practice. An example, though, is that if your practice averages 1,000 patient visits per month, an incentive threshold might be a 10% increase. Granted, that's if your practice is capable of handling the increased volume without compromising quality. And, as mentioned before, if that's your goal, you need to provide the employee with the tools for bringing about that increase, whether it's marketing suggestions or an increased marketing budget.

R-E-S-P-E-C-T

Our experience from traveling throughout the US and talking with medical assistants is that money, surprisingly, is not necessarily at the top of their list of motivators. Asking them the question, "What motivates you the most at work?" the answers we get the most are "sense of fulfillment," "respect" or "employer gratitude."

> *"Ownership has to do with the employee's ability to take personal responsibility and accountability for producing results."*

Another common motivator is ownership. That isn't to say they own the practice, but that they have ownership of their job, the freedom to do it well, the acknowledgement of when they do it well, and the feeling that what they do matters, both to you and the patients. Ownership has to do with the employee's ability to take personal responsibility and accountability for producing results.

Nonfinancial rewards are tricky, since they're not necessarily linked to money. They are linked to a philosophy and that philosophy has to come from you. In our opinion, terms such as "Thank you" and "Good job" are the most forgotten forms of reward. We believe that a financial incentive that is not integrated into a nonfinancial program is likely to fail. Examples are:

- A sincere thank you. Don't take your staff for granted.
- Public acknowledgements, such as an "Employee of the month" award. Or, we suppose, some sort of Cracker Jack Award.
- Private acknowledgements. That can be a Post-it® note saying "Good job" or a private email, or a moment in the hallway or your office when you say, "You did a good job. Thank you."
- A hybrid incentive. It can be a small gift like movie tickets or a gift certificate.

Some of this comes down to philosophy. Tom Peters, in his book *A Passion for Excellence*, challenges his readers to make fundamental changes in the way they interact with employees. There is a tendency for bosses to look for things that are wrong. Peters charged readers to "catch them doing something right." It's all too easy as a manager to habitually criticize, which can lead to a destructive attitude on the part of employees who then decide that since they can't do anything right, they shouldn't bother trying.

Your staff is your practice's most important asset. Keep them motivated, fulfilled and enthused using a combination of financial and nonfinancial incentives.

Action Step: Plan 1 motivational action for (each employee this month) each of the next 3 months. List the 10 simple things you can do to motivate and thank your office team.

The Paperless Office

Electronic medical records, digital equipment and health information technology.

A revolution has struck the medical office in the last decade, and it's the concept of the paperless office. That is to say, not only are practitioners using computers, but they are fully utilizing electronic medical records (EMR), electronic health records (EHR), electronic office software for transcription and charting, automated scheduling software, automated appointment reminders, digital x-ray, ultrasound and fluoroscopes, and digital prescription software.

This section is not meant to be comprehensive, but rather to provide an overview of options and present some of the considerations a physician must make before deciding which digital products to implement.

ONLINE APPOINTMENT SCHEDULING

These systems are typically linked to your practice's Web site—you do have a Web site, right? Once on the Web site, there is a button that says something like: To Make An Online Appointment. The patient inputs his or her own information and is provided a password. The patient doesn't get to see the physician schedule, but they are provided option dates with the physician that they can then schedule. Typically, the schedule is controlled by someone on staff, such as your office manager. The staffer inputs a time block for the physician. The patient picks the time and the appointment is confirmed via email. The software often is designed to generate an automatic reminder.

Some of the advantages to this is it decreases telephone time for one of your staffers. In addition, you as a physician can access your schedule from anywhere in the world. Many patients, at least the more tech-savvy ones, often like it because they feel more in control.

The online appointment scheduling system can also be linked to online billing inquiries, so your staff can research billing problems before getting back with the patient instead of placing the patient on hold or interrupting their workflow to handle a question.

> *"Some physicians don't like these systems because they set a different tone than having a patient talk to a friendly receptionist."*

Some perks of these systems is the ability to do blast emails to all of your patients. This can become part of your marketing campaign, as well as a way of offering new services or new products. Some physicians don't like these systems because they set a different tone than having a patient talk to a friendly receptionist.

ONLINE BILLING AND INSURANCE CONFIRMATION

A number of companies that offer online scheduling also offer billing software. One example is NueMD, offered by Nuesoft Technologies, Inc. This software connects your in-office computer to the company's mainframe, which can handle your billing needs as well as online insurance eligibility verification. An excellent source for lists of goods and services is *www.mpmbuyersguide.com*.

Again, this can save your staff time otherwise spent on the phone with insurance companies. It places you, the physician, in control of buying and installing the system, but puts training, upgrading, and HIPAA and insurance compliance on the shoulders of the software provider. Many also provide daily data backups.

ELECTRONIC MEDICAL RECORDS AND ELECTRONIC HEALTH RECORDS

Electronic medical records (EMR) and electronic health records (EHR) are often used interchangeably. However, the government doesn't do this and defines them separately. An EMR is essentially a legal record created in hospitals or ambulatory medical environments involving medical information. An EMR is the source material for an EHR. An EHR is defined as a personal health record (also sometimes called a PHR) in digital form.

In 2005, the US Department of Health and Human Services (DHHS) awarded a contract to the Certification Commission for Healthcare Information Technology (CCHIT) to certify EMRs and EHRs. If either product is not certified by CCHIT, stay away, because certification assures that the system you've invested in can interact with any government-based health records that may come into play in the future. Also, the federal government has put a number of incentives into place to encourage utilization of EMRs and EHRs, but in order to benefit from those incentives the system needs government approval.

E-PRESCRIBING

E-prescribing is a computer program that creates a document that writes a prescription. These programs are either standalone or, increasingly, part of an EMR. The physician can fill out a patient drug prescription on the computer and it gets sent directly to the patient's pharmacy. Nothing gets written by hand and the patients do not need to deliver the prescription themselves.

E-prescribing will be dealt with in more detail in Essential #15.

> **Action Step:** Take steps this month (trade shows, online, etc) to perform due diligence on EHR implementation. Create a simple written plan on how you are planning to begin EHR usage. Set goals relating to this with a timeline and stick to it!

ESSENTIAL #14:

Remote Access

"I'll have an office—and I'll take it to go."
Working from home or on the road.

The Internet is a wonderful thing. It has revolutionized the world, how we entertain ourselves, how we do business.

For physicians, you can now access your notes and medical records from anywhere in the world—at your home or on the road. If you have multiple office sites, you can operate 1 office IT system that can be accessed from the other site. A physician is, after all, a mobile worker. Your job doesn't entail sitting in an office all day. You're in with patients, you're in your office, you're at the hospital, you're on the road.

The obvious way to do this is via laptops or desktop computers at your location. However, a growing trend is the use of smartphones like the iPhone or the Android. Smartphones are essentially mobile telephones with computer-like functionality. That functionality typically includes email, Internet access, and some sort of screen and keyboard that allows for an interface—the touchscreen interface is growing in popularity due to the iPhone, but some people prefer keyboards.

In addition, there is a growth in tablet computers, with the Apple iPad possibly being a game-changer in this arena, allowing larger screen real estate to do more web surfing and have access to larger images. Netbooks, which are smaller and less expensive (and less powerful, generally speaking) are also a possibility.

Because the iPhone Enterprise Platform was so inexpensive—a standard program license costs $99 and for companies with 500 or more employees it is $299—everybody with a little programming skill and an idea started writing programs that could be used on the iPhone. Some of those—a growing number—are health and medicine related.

There are about 8 different smartphone platforms: Android (Google), BlackBerry, iPhone, iPod Touch, Nokia Symbian, Palm OS, Palm Pre classic and Windows Mobile. Although the iPhone kicked off the rush for smartphone-related programs, more competitive companies began developing multiple-platform software.

There are literally hundreds of programs available for physicians. Here is a partial list of interesting applications:

- **Epocrates, Inc.** (*www.epocrates.com*)
  Epocrates offers a variety of different apps for smartphones, including their free Epocrates Rx, a handheld drug reference that provides information about each drug, adverse reactions, contraindications, drug interactions and pricing.
- **Caretools** (*www.caretools.com*)
  Caretools, developed by a physician (Dr. Thomas Giannulli, MD, MS) for physicians, offers an app called iChart, which includes iPrescribing, iBilling, iLab Reports and iNotes.

They encrypt their entire database, requiring a password and PIN code for accessing information, and are completely HIPAA compliant.

- **QxMD** (*www.qxmd.com*)

   Founded by Dr. Daniel Schwartz, MD, QxMD produces a number of different programs aimed at physicians, including Cardio Calc, The ECG Guide, QxMD ICD-9 Coder, GI Calc, Heme Cal, Neph Calc and many others, including translation programs for Cantonese and Mandarin.

- **Skyscape, Inc.** (*www.skyscape.com*)

   Skyscape has more than 500 products geared toward 35 medical specialties and has a registered user base of more than 12 million practitioners. They provide drug resources, laboratory and diagnostics databases and references, medical calculators and medical news. Some of their products are *ACC Pocket Guide—Management of Patients With Chronic Stable Angina, Archimedes Online (Medical Calculator)* and *ACCF Pocket Guidelines.*

> *"Epocrates conducted a study looking at time savings,*
> *which concluded that 50% of their users saved 20 minutes or*
> *more every day using their software applications."*

The use of these devices, which can have a kind of gee-whiz quality to them, are actually proving to increase physician efficiency. Epocrates conducted a study looking at time savings, which concluded that 50% of their users saved 20 minutes or more every day using their software applications. Much of those savings had to do with avoiding pharmacy callbacks and being able to look up information while with the patient vs leaving the examining room.

SECURITY

Of course, there are always going to be security issues when it comes to accessing patient records using the Internet. Both HIPAA and the Health Information Technology for Economic and Clinical Health (HITECH) Act have placed more emphasis—and penalties—on security breaches. Some of these are very specific to remote access and mobile devices:

1. *Device and Media Control. (164.310(d)(1)).* This refers to any device used in the practice, as well as to devices like flash drives (or pin drives, or thumb drivers, whatever they're being called). It's entirely too easy for someone on staff to use a flash drive to access confidential medical records and take them with them; or vice versa, bring in something from home that may have malware such as viruses or spyware in it. One solution is to lock up the computers' USB ports or have a strong policy in place letting employees know this behavior will not be tolerated. This can be a problem with a smartphone if any patient data is stored in its memory or there are no access controls.

2. *Access Control. (164.312(a)(1).* Access control, similar to Workstation Use, applies to the security protocols put into place for access to your system. There are 2 components. One

is logging in from the desktop and the other is remote access. If someone, a physician or office manager, is logging into the system from a remote location, there needs to be a secure connection, but also, the home computer's security and connection needs to be checked to make sure they're not bringing in viruses or spyware. They also need to assure their wi-fi connection is not an open conduit to every neighbor or passing hacker.

3. *Person or Entity Authentication (164.312(d))*. Related to access control, it refers to making sure that the person who is accessing the system is actually the person they say they are. This can apply to background checks on new hires, as well. Physicians are a major target for identity theft because of the wealth of information on their systems. In fact, one of the sheriff's departments in New Jersey has a task force that is a splinter of their gang task force. All they do is investigate cyber crimes against physicians. They have found that gangs are now looking at identity theft because it's so lucrative, and it's easier and less risky than selling drugs and other traditional gang-related activities.

4. *Transmission Security (164.312(3)(1)*. Transmission security refers to making certain your practice's server is locked down and that security protocols are in place.

So although it's clear that remote access and mobile devices can be a real boon to a busy doctor, they are not without risks and hazards.

Note: Ray Posa, CEO of The Manta Group, assisted with this chapter.

Action Step: List ways in which technology might enhance your out-of-the-office productivity. What new systems do you want to implement to increase efficiency and save time when away from the office? Can any of this technology help anyone else on your office team?

ESSENTIAL #15:

E-prescribing

Reaping the rewards of e-prescribing systems.

In 2006, the Institute of Medicine published a study finding that, in the US, about 7,000 deaths are caused each year by medication errors. For some perspective on that number, imagine a 747 jet crashing every month for a year and having no survivors. Or imagine two 9/11 terrorist events.

E-prescribing can help solve those medication errors. Interestingly, a study put out in 2010 by SureScripts, the leading e-prescribing service, found that only 1 in 4 office-based physicians were using e-prescribing.

> *"In 2006, the Institute of Medicine published a study finding that, in the US, about 7,000 deaths are caused each year by medication errors. For some perspective on that number, imagine a 747 jet crashing every month for a year and having no survivors. Or imagine two 9/11 terrorist events."*

WHAT IS IT?

E-prescribing is a computer program that allows a physician to fill a patient drug prescription on the computer; it is then sent directly to the patient's pharmacy. Nothing handwritten is involved and, in most cases, the patients don't need to deliver the prescription themselves. They just go to their local pharmacy where the prescription was directed and pick up their medicine.

The programs are either standalone or part of an electronic medical record. Although individual programs vary, many allow the physician to set up a list of common drugs and dosages, as well as generic alternatives. Also, many e-prescribing programs automatically confirm the patient's insurance formulary—no more phone tag with the pharmacy. Just imagine how much office staff time that saves!

Medicare Part D's prescription drug program defines e-prescribing as the following:

> *"E-prescribing means the transmission, using electronic media, of prescription or prescription-related information between a prescriber, dispenser, pharmacy benefit manager, or health plan, either directly or through an intermediary, including an e-prescribing network. E-prescribing includes, but is not limited to, two-way transmissions between the point of care and the dispenser."*

This definition also includes, as of 2003, electronic faxes from the physician's office to the pharmacy (although the fax method is losing favor to an all-electronic information exchange).

A LITTLE TECHNICAL BACKGROUND

Like the banking industry and ATMs, e-prescribing doesn't quite travel over the general purpose Internet. E-prescribing has an IT backbone that securely channels connections between prescribers, pharmacies and pharmaceutical benefit managers. In 2001, two separate companies essentially ran that backbone—SureScripts and RxHub. In July 2008, they combined to become SureScripts-RxHub.

SureScripts was formed by the pharmacy industry—the National Association of Chain Drug Stores (NACDS) and the National Community Pharmacists Association (NCPA)—with the plan to develop a network that would handle the electronic exchange of prescription information between physician practices and pharmacies.

RxHub was formed by the 3 biggest pharmaceutical benefit managers (PBMs)—CVS Caremark Corporation, Express Scripts, Inc. and Medco Health Solutions. Their task was to deliver prescription benefit information from the big PBMs to physician practices—delivery of formularies, benefit eligibility and medication history information.

The joint company makes money in 2 basic ways. The major PBMs pay a transaction fee to deliver their formulary prescription benefit information. And pharmacists pay a transaction fee when they receive a prescription. Physicians don't get charged anything; in fact, SureScripts-RxHub pays physicians a small fee. The extent of a physician's expenses for using e-prescribing has to do with whatever program they buy or acquire (because some programs are free).

3 E-PRESCRIBING OPTIONS

There are (at least) 3 approaches to e-prescribing.
1. *Standalone.* This isn't quite as popular as it might have been for several reasons. First, most physicians want some sort of EMR, and many EMRs have e-prescribing built in or available as a module. Second, there are ongoing Medicare incentive programs (see below) that require EHRs be interoperable with other EHRs that require an e-prescribing system.
2. *Part of an EMR.* As mentioned above, many EMRs have e-prescribing built in. Allscripts is one of the leading clinical software providers, used by about a third of all doctors in the US (about 155,000, as well as 700 hospitals and 5,000 extended care facilities). An e-prescribing program is part of the EMR product.
3. *Free!* For someone wanting to jump into e-prescribing without any up-front costs, primarily as a way to get your feet wet, the National ePrescribing Patient Safety Initiative (NEPSI), which was founded by Allscripts, Dell and other companies, including

Microsoft, Google and Fujitsu, offers a free downloadable e-prescription program on their Web site: *http://www.nationalerx.com*.

E-prescribing systems range from free (NEPSI) to about $2,500 per year. According to the Congressional Budget Office, more complicated EHR systems range in price from about $25,000–$45,000 per physician. Operating and maintaining those systems, including software licensing fees, tech support and upgrades, is estimated to range between $3,000–$9,000 per physician per year. Those prices are easily offset by overall efficiency, and current government incentives more than pay for them.

ADVANTAGES

It doesn't require a lot of thought to see the advantages to e-prescribing. Efficiency is one of the first, of course. Phone calls and call-backs to pharmacies are, at the very least, decreased, and often almost completely eliminated. Faxes will be minimized, and prescription renewal and authorization can be automated. Some e-prescribing systems even allow the physician's staff to pull in medication history as part of the process.

Patient convenience is another advantage. The patient no longer needs to drop off a prescription at their pharmacy and wait for it or come back for it. Many physicians believe this results in greater patient compliance.

E-prescribing systems can reference a patient's formulary, which saves time and hassle for physicians and their staff—no guessing games to figure out what drugs are on formulary.

And as mentioned at the beginning of the chapter, most studies indicate that e-prescribing will dramatically decrease medication errors.

INCENTIVES

Starting in January 2009, Medicare started offering financial incentives to physicians using a qualified e-prescribing system. A qualified system had 4 requirements:

1. It had to be able to generate a complete active medication list that incorporated electronic data from applicable pharmacy drug plans, if available;
2. It had to be able to select medications, print prescriptions, electronically transmit prescriptions and conduct all safety checks, which include automated prompts that provide drug description, potential inappropriate dosage or administration routes, drug-drug interactions, drug-allergy interactions, or any other warnings or cautions;
3. It had to provide information concerning the availability of a lower cost, therapeutically appropriate alternative drug, if available;
4. It needed to provide information on formulary or tiered formulary medications, a patient's eligibility and authorization requirements received electronically from the patient's drug plan.

There's no indication these carrots and sticks are going away, so there are many reasons for physicians to jump into using an e-prescribing system. A number of states have also created initiatives.

CONTROLLED SUBSTANCE ISSUES

One problem with e-prescriptions is the DEA's prohibition against electronic transmission for prescriptions for controlled substances. According to the AMA, about 20% of prescriptions are for controlled substances. So in these cases, the e-prescription program prints out the prescription and the physician must manually sign it. The printer must also be kept in a secure area. The EHR or e-prescription program can still be used to generate and document the prescription, but it needs to be printed and signed.

The DEA issued a proposal in July 2008 to allow controlled substances to be e-prescribed. In the March 31, 2010 issue of the Federal Register, they issued an interim rule that allowed electronic transmission of controlled substance prescriptions.

CONSIDERATIONS

We think there are 7 things physicians should consider before implementing an e-prescribing system.

1. Decide if you want a full EMR or just e-prescribing. Is your practice ready for a full EMR?
2. What do you think will cause your practice the most problems? Best to implement a little at a time if your staff has problems adapting to major change.
3. Get everyone involved. Everybody needs to learn how this system works, physician included.
4. Think through your workflow. What are the implications of switching from paper to electronic medication management? How will your staff have to change and adapt?
5. What kind of hardware? What are you using now and what has to change to make this work?
6. Train appropriately. Prepare yourself and your staff for the training time and expertise that's needed to make an e-prescribing system work effectively. Anticipate what problems your staff and patients will encounter and how you might deal with them.
7. Tell your patients about it.

Action Step: Investigate, set up and utilize e-prescribing within the next 6 months. Write a timeline and steps necessary for the implementation and decide who on your office team will be responsible for each step.

Billing Company Or In-house Billing?

The pros and cons of handling billing yourself or hiring a billing firm.

The decision of whether to handle your billing in-house or hire a billing company is not trivial. Typically, a billing company takes 6%–9% of the monies they handle, which is a significant chunk of change. If your practice handles $1 million annually, that amounts to $60,000–$90,000. If you can handle billing yourself and do it well, the costs can drop to about 3% of monies, or $30,000. Given the opportunity to save $30,000–$60,000 annually, most physicians would take it. But it may not be that simple a decision.

It really comes down to whether the practitioner has a fundamental knowledge of coding, billing and collecting. If you don't, it's better to outsource.

CONS

First, be aware that, in addition to the percentage a billing company charges, they typically charge a set-up fee that ranges anywhere from $500–$3,000. One of the effects of that is it makes it unlikely you'll jump to a competing billing company, because you'll have to lay out the fee again.

Billing companies also often lock you into a contract for a specific period of time. Breaking the contract if you weren't happy with the service requires that you prove they are not measuring up to industry standards. Industry standards, unfortunately, aren't all that stringent or well established.

Many billing companies, like help desks, outsource their work overseas. Troubleshooting may require you spending time on an international phone call at your expense with someone whose grasp of English is limited or made more difficult with a heavy accent.

Some billing services are set up so the checks are sent directly to them, rather than to you. The company then disperses the money after they take their fees out. This is one area we strongly advise against, because you totally lose control over your funds, even before you know if the company performs satisfactorily.

> *"One of the most common complaints about billing services is that they don't chase the money. They are paid on a percentage, so they put their time into handling bigger customers and/or bigger claims. That's simple math: Get 7% of $1,000 or 7% of $10,000. They chase the low-hanging fruit rather than claims that are more challenging."*

One of the most common complaints about billing services is that they don't chase the money. They are paid on a percentage, so they put their time into handling bigger customers and/or bigger claims. That's simple math: Get 7% of $1,000 or 7% of $10,000. They chase the low-hanging fruit rather than claims that are more challenging.

Another problem is that billing for various specialties has its own difficulties and quirks, its own codes. If you opt for a billing company, check for references and make sure it has experience working with your specialty.

PROS

Granted, both of us do our own billing in-house, so we're biased toward it. But one of the real difficulties in doing your own billing is that it's complicated and constantly changing. To do your own billing—which in reality means you need at least 1 skilled person on your staff to do this—you not only have to be educated in it, but continue to stay up-to-date on billing procedures, attend seminars regularly, and keep up on coding changes and modifiers. It's an ongoing learning process.

Billing is not taught in medical school. As a new practitioner, you are going to have to go out on your own and hire a billing company anyway just to get started. Otherwise, the learning curve is huge, and you're already at a point in your career where you're learning many new things. It's much easier to hire a billing service at that point. As you get well versed in billing, then you can take it in-house.

If you send billing out, that frees up your staff for other duties. Hal does his own billing, but he has 4 full-time billing personnel, which is a fairly heavy personnel component of the practice.

A professional billing service can streamline your billing processes. And if you have a professional, high-quality billing company that you trust, it can eliminate a lot of headaches and concerns. You need to balance the costs of the billing service with the costs of training and employing the people you have doing billing in-house.

Many billing companies have certified coders and billers.

"If a patient calls up with a problem about billing, you're still the one that needs to solve it for the patient, even if you're demanding an explanation from your billing company. It all starts with the doctor."

Ignorance, by the way, is not acceptable. You, as a physician, still have responsibilities concerning billing. You have to make sure that whatever you're circling on the chart and sending off to the billing company is accurate. If a patient calls up with a problem about billing, you're still the one that needs to solve it for the patient, even if you're demanding an explanation from your billing company. It all starts with the doctor.

CONSIDERATIONS

Let's assume that you've decided to hire a billing company. What do you need to think about?

First, is the company familiar with your specialty? Are they familiar with the intricacies of the codes and modifiers that are necessary for your specialty? Do they have other clients in the same specialty? We absolutely recommend asking for references to speak with those clients.

Second, are you required to purchase software that integrates with the billing company? That exact cost has to be accounted for.

Third, do you have access to your accounts? Can you go online and review the accounts as they stand with the billing and collection company?

Fourth, determine exactly what the billing company is going to do. The contract must specify the exact duties the company will perform. Are they going to submit claims? Are they going to get involved in collecting claims? If they are going to be involved in collections, are they going to get involved in patient receivables as well as insurance receivables? The billing and collections firm's contract must spell out exactly what services they will do for the money you're paying.

Fifth, be aware that many billing services get complacent. Don't assume they know what's going on. You need to be able to track what the billing company is doing. Ask if you can access your own records. Is it by request or do they have an online access system?

Sixth, what are the billing company's procedures? What is their billing protocol? In other words, what is their action play when a claim is 30 days old? 60? 90? 120? They should be able to provide you with a detailed action plan for what happens at each one of these steps. They can't just wait for a claim to be 90 days old before they take action on it. We also recommend that you provide the billing company with a written document that indicates what you believe the action steps are that should be taken for each stage of the process.

Seventh, ask the billing company what their average *days in receivables* is. This tells you how long the average claim floats in the ether before it gets paid. It's a good indicator of how good the company is at collecting claims.

Eighth, make sure you fully understand the billing service's termination requirements in the contract. If you don't like them, ask them to change the requirements or don't sign it. Termination requirements should protect the practitioner as well as the billing company.

Ninth, ask if they outsource services or if everything is performed in-office.

Tenth, if the billing company requires office software, ask about installation, troubleshooting and upgrades.

Eleventh, ask if the billing service's staff are certified as coders/billers.

Twelfth, ask about the billing service's continuing education and how they stay up-to-date on changes in billing and coding.

Above all, ask questions and don't make a decision until you're satisfied with the answers.

Action Step: Measure and monitor billing/collections strengths and weaknesses quarterly and compare to industry benchmarks. List pros and cons of switching the way you do billing (in-house vs a billing service) and if there is a significant reason for changing. If so, list action items for possible change.

Seven Practice Assessments

Financial soundness, overhead expenses, managed care costs, patient encounters, services, product, client satisfaction.

Once your practice is up and running—or if it's been up and running for a while—it's a good idea to regularly ask yourself: How am I doing? If the patients come in and leave happy and satisfied, if money is getting made, bills are getting paid and your staff seem content with their jobs, from 20,000 feet it looks like things are going well.

But it's a good idea to use objective standards to regularly find out if your practice is really doing well, or even if it's doing as well as you think it is. There may be some leaks you're unaware of: Your practice could be doing better or could be headed for trouble.

To understand your practice, you need to know what your practice is. The benchmarks for a plastic surgery practice are not the same for a dentist, a family practitioner or a podiatrist. In addition, within your specialty, do you know what your subspecialty is? For instance, if you are a dentist, are you in general dentistry? Do you focus on children? If you're a podiatrist, do you focus on the diabetic patient? On athletic medicine? On gerontology?

Knowing what you want your practice to be helps define how you're doing in terms of achieving those goals.

A corollary to that is: What do your patients want?

A patient's needs will vary, depending not only on your specialty, but your subspecialty. This helps to focus the goals of your practice. It's a somewhat soft type of benchmarking, where the focus isn't on financial figures, but on patient satisfaction. If you can determine what patients want, you can determine whether you're providing it. You can then determine the best ways to provide that care.

PRACTICE ASSESSMENTS

There are 7 practice assessments that should be analyzed when considering overall benchmarks. They are:

1. *Financial Soundness.* These include gross charges, net collections, accounts receivable, debt-to-equity ratios and current assets to current liabilities.
2. *Overhead Expenses.* Overhead expenses include occupancy costs (rent or mortgage), equipment, supplies, staff and benefits.
3. *Managed Care Costs.* These include capitation rates, quality assurance and utilization management issues.
4. *Patient Encounters.* How many patients do you see daily? How many new patients? How many encounters per physician per full-time equivalent (FTE)?

5. *Services.* These include subcontracted or subcapitated services or carve-outs, ancillary services, outsourcing, and costs of services calculated through activity-based costing or other methods. Basically, anything you hire to be done or send out to be performed.
6. *Product.* This includes revenue per hour, encounters per hour, encounters per procedure, revenues per FTE and payer mix.
7. *Client Satisfaction.* Besides a more general sense of client satisfaction, you need to look at assessing client satisfaction by segregating patients by type of insurance and studying your rate of patient turnover.

These are all categories that should be considered when actually looking at benchmarks; then you need to decide which categories you want—or need—to analyze.

"All benchmarks are not created equal. As a result,
some of them are more important than others."

BENCHMARKS

All benchmarks are not created equal. As a result, some of them are more important than others. For instance, many physicians place great stock in the number of new patients. Others may focus on how many patients are seen.

Per Visit Value

We think a significantly more important benchmark is the per visit value (PVV). The PVV is determined by dividing total collections by total patient visits:

(Total Collections/Total Patient Visits = Per Visit Value)

The average PVV will vary depending on specialty. For instance, in podiatry, the number you see cited the most is $99, although some sources cite $90.

Although this is a very basic benchmark, it's one that has ramifications in every type of business, whether it's an online business (Per Click Value) or a restaurant (Per Customer Value), etc. PVV provides a value of how productive you are.

However, because we're physicians, it doesn't always come down to a dollar amount. You need to look at what you're doing for each patient—not just injections, not just visits or ancillary care, but vascular testing, neurological testing, physical therapy in your office and dispensing products in-office.

Payroll Ratio

Payroll ratio is calculated by taking your total staff payroll—not just salary of support staff, but the salaries and payroll taxes and benefits, like 401Ks, and totaling them (for just the support staff)—and dividing that number by annual collections. This provides the payroll ratio and, if your practice is operating efficiently, it should be somewhere between 22%–26% of collections.

$$\text{(Total Staff Payroll/Annual Collections} = \text{Payroll Ratio)}$$

Accounts Receivable

Accounts receivable (A/R) will also vary from practice specialty to practice specialty, but one rule of thumb is that a practice's total accounts receivable is <2 months worth of gross charges. For example, if your practice is billing $65,000 per month, the practice should have a total A/R of less than $130,000. In addition, you will want <15% of the total accounts receivable to be 90 days outstanding.

This particular benchmark can be taken one step further, to *days in receivables*, which is defined as how long the average claim takes to be paid. The equation for that is:

$$\text{([Total Accounts Receivable/Gross Annual Charges] X 365}$$
$$= \text{Days in Receivables)}$$

Miscellaneous

There are a number of benchmarks a physician can use to get a handle on how their practice is doing. One is simply to track trends—are new patients increasing or decreasing, for instance.

- Is the volume of x-rays increasing or decreasing?
- Is the volume of sutures increasing or decreasing?
- Is the volume of injections increasing or decreasing?

It can be done with almost anything in your practice, but the key is to then superimpose the data, which is where practice management software can come in handy. How do these relate to each other? Do new patients require more x-rays?

If the practice management software you use is capable of capturing diagnoses, and patients by diagnoses, that provides useful information. For example, you can benchmark the injections with the diagnosis of injections. You can benchmark x-rays for the diagnoses that apply to x-rays.

DRAWBACKS TO BENCHMARKS

Each individual practice specialty has different benchmarks. Typically, the specialty's professional organization, such as the American Academy of Family Physicians or the American Academy of Podiatric Practice Management, conducts regular surveys that then become the yardstick that you measure your practice against. The problem with this is that there is often an inherent problem with these surveys—they report average or median values. You want your practice to be the best, or Best of Class (BOC), not "average," which often means mediocre.

"Although numbers are useful measures of your
practice's success, they don't necessarily measure what's
most important: Patient satisfaction."

And although numbers are useful measures of your practice's success, they don't necessarily measure what's most important: Patient satisfaction. There are potentially 3 questions that need to be asked that have nothing to do with numbers:

1. Are you improving patient care?
2. Are you improving your quality of life?
3. Are you increasing the bottom line?

Patient satisfaction is Number One. But other questions that are important are: Are you, the physician, happy? Are you fulfilled? Is your profession doing for you what you thought it should or want it to?

Too often, the answer is: No.

But perhaps, if they took the time to look at their practice data and figure out how to interpret the numbers, then physicians would become empowered to respond appropriately and turn their practice—and their fulfillment—around.

The question is: How is your practice doing?

Hopefully, the answer is: Better than yesterday, and we're going to try and make it better tomorrow.

> **Action Step:** Monitor your practice data monthly, quarterly and annually. Create simple spreadsheets for assessment and identify areas of concern. Write action plans for improvement. Appoint appropriate team members to help with each of these areas.

ESSENTIAL #18:

Controlling Overhead

**_Don't get eaten alive! Evaluating and controlling your costs,
including salaries, benefits and other expenses._**

A business can raise revenue in 2 ways: Increase business or cut costs. Although much of this book deals with direct and indirect ways to increase revenue and run your practice efficiently, attention needs to be paid to controlling overhead. Over the last 15 years, most group practices have reported that costs have risen 35% or more, but revenue has only increased by about 21%. That's seriously out of whack.

FIRST THINGS FIRST

You can't start slashing your budget until you know exactly how much you're spending and what you're spending on. You really need to drill down into your profit/loss (P/L) statement and find the details, or *granularity*, as the business-speak folks like to say.

Most medical practices' P/L statements don't provide enough detail. This can cause no end of trouble when trying to determine where to cut. For example, often the category that is largest—salary—seems like the first place to start cutting. That may be true, but by creating more detailed "buckets," or line items, you can get a more nuanced approach to budget cutting.

Another example is "supplies." That simply does not provide enough detail to be useful. There needs to be subcategories, such as "medical supplies" and "administrative supplies" and so on.

Salaries, then, isn't accurate: You need staff benefits, staff salaries, payroll taxes, education expenses, overtime. Once you have your categories broken down, it's much easier to compare expenses and overhead against national benchmarks for your practice's specialty areas. If your practice spends more than others in your specialty area on specific line items like salaries, supplies or rent, then you can analyze those line items to determine why that is.

Granted, national averages are not necessarily the most useful indicator of your expenses, but can point to areas that may be problematic. There also may be very good reasons for your specific areas to be higher than the national average. Perhaps you offer extended hours or perform a great deal of emergency care, resulting in higher staff expenses. Alternately, the type of care you offer may result in higher revenue per volume than other practices.

*"National averages are not necessarily the most useful indicator of your
expenses, but can point to areas that may be problematic."*

7 OBVIOUS CHOICES FOR A FIRST LOOK

Although these aren't the only areas you can look at to cut costs, they're the first you should look at and where cutting back won't put your practice in trouble.

1. *Malpractice insurance discounts.* Look for discounts for your malpractice insurance. Some carriers offer discounts for practices that attend a risk management course or for using EMRs. Shop around and see if you can find lower rates from competitors.

2. *Evaluate advertising costs.* Too many physicians approach advertising and marketing as if it were pasta—they fling it at the wall and see what sticks. But you can save a lot of money and time by researching your marketing plan, using measurable metrics to evaluate return on investment (ROI) and creating a plan, rather than a series of random advertisements and promotional events.

3. *Buy in bulk.* Monitoring your inventory is important. Don't buy too much, which ties up capital, but not having enough can hurt the efficiency of your practice and increase shipping charges. Try to negotiate for better deals with competing vendors. Also, make sure that billable supplies get reimbursed appropriately—they should at least equal their costs!

4. *Evaluate your phone service.* Telephone companies want your business and are often willing to negotiate better prices to get it. Evaluate Voice Over Internet Protocol (VoIP) options and bundled phone and cable Internet services to bring down prices. Not only should you analyze your phone bills and look for trends and usage patterns, but let competing phone carriers analyze your existing call patterns and volume. They may offer you a better service package.

5. *Evaluate services and equipment.* Medical practices often hire a variety of services, from cleaning services to billing or accounting services. Are they doing a good job? Are they giving you a good deal? Can some of these be brought in-house effectively for less money? The key word there is *effectively.* You don't want to derail your staff's efficiency by overloading them with tasks that can be done better by outside firms. Still, some services can be divvied up efficiently—perhaps outsource payroll, but have someone in-house responsible for accounts payable.

6. *Do a lease-vs-buy analysis of equipment.* Assumptions about overall costs for equipment can come back to bite you. Are you sure buying equipment was the right approach? Did you have to replace it or upgrade it 2 years later? Sometimes outright purchase can be better than leasing, but not always. Working with your accountant to evaluate the numbers can help you make the best decision.

7. *Take a hard look at your facility.* Is your ego getting in the way? Is your office too big? Can you share an office? Are exam rooms being used to capacity? Is there storage space going unused? Or not enough storage space? Can some space be used more effectively for in-office dispensing, displays of durable medical equipment or other ancillary products? Are you running a satellite office? Is it cost effective or is it bleeding dollars?

ASK YOUR STAFF

Ask your staff if they can think of ways to cut costs. Have a brainstorming session and see what they come up with. They will want to protect salaries and benefits, so they may become very creative in coming up with efficiencies that may not be obvious to you. It also helps create ownership in the practice, knowing that their decisions and involvement will improve the practice's overall health.

Action Step: List 5 strategies that will reduce your expenses over the next 12 months. Blend these strategies together with the Action Step from Essential #3, and make sure they become part of your budget projections.

ESSENTIAL #19:

Ancillary Services

The comprehensive and collaborative care model.
Offering physical therapy or other secondary services.

The 2 most obvious ways to increase revenue are to work longer hours and see more patients, or to cut staff. These are not necessarily desirable. First, a physician can only work so many hours before it cuts into their quality of life, and second, cutting staff may make it more difficult to see patients.

Many physicians look to adding ancillary services as a way to increase revenue. Possible ancillary services will vary depending on specialty, but options include:

- Anesthesia
- Antiaddiction centers
- Antiaging centers
- Catheterization laboratories
- Diabetes and weight management programs
- Diagnostic testing
- Dialysis centers
- Endoscopy centers
- Freestanding ambulatory surgery centers (ASCs)
- Geriatric centers
- Infusion therapy centers
- Pain management
- Physical therapy
- Psychotherapy centers
- Retail product sales, such as eyeglasses, hearing aids, orthotics, etc.
- Skin care centers
- Sleep centers
- Urgent care centers
- Weight loss centers
- Wellness centers
- X-ray services laboratories

There are many things to consider before jumping into ancillary services. One of the first simply is: Will it improve patient care?

Other important factors are your own ability and willingness to supervise the delivery of the ancillary services.

Let's break it down into 10 considerations:

1. **What ancillary services are you currently ordering out?** If you or, if you're in a group practice, your fellow physicians, routinely refer patients to other locations for basic lab work, x-rays, PET scans, physical therapy, etc, then those are prime targets for your own ancillary service offerings. An addendum to that is, if it were available within your office, would you be more likely to order it for a patient? It has to, of course, be medically appropriate, so tamp down excess optimism you might have about getting rich off your in-office laboratory.

2. **What are up-front ancillary equipment costs?** These could be called "hard assets." Is there a lot of equipment involved in your proposed ancillary service? Can it be bought or leased? Can it be bought used? Identify the costs for equipment, software, fixtures, etc. Consider financing options, talk to a vendor and your bank. Discussing this with your practice management consultant or an accountant with experience in this area will help to identify hard expenses you may not be aware of.

3. **What are ancillary support costs?** Having calculated the hard costs, now look at space, personnel and management costs. Will the ancillary service be offered within your existing practice space or at a new location? Will you have to make changes to your existing structure to accommodate the new service? Do you need new staff? What are staffing needs? Will they be full-time or part-time? Will current staff require additional training? Does the new service require a different type of management system or resources, whether financial or operational? Can your staff handle it from a training perspective, or time and efficiency perspective? Would it make sense to hire a third-party manager to handle the new service?

4. **Third-party approval and regulatory issues?** Many ancillary services require licensing. Some of that licensing will be done by the state, some by the federal government. Accreditation may be required before you can be reimbursed; some insurers and third-party payers will reimburse at a higher level if your ancillary service is approved by an accreditation body. Not only is this time consuming, but it can be expensive.

   A laboratory, for instance, needs to be licensed by the Clinical Laboratory Improvement Amendments (CLIA), part of the Department of Health and Human Services. Licensure depends on the types of tests being performed—waived vs non-waived (or low-complexity vs medium- to high-complexity)—and the fees and director certifications vary. And not only that, but regular inspections and compliance issues are involved as well.

5. **Figure out how much you can charge.** An ancillary service is a business and you need to understand that business—how much money can it bring in, who pays, how much? As in most businesses, in order to determine what you can charge, you need historical data. Typically professional organizations or other practitioners with the same ancillary services should be able to provide that information. The information

should also be compared by payors. Once you have the possible number of referrals and the potential reimbursement, you can project revenue.

6. **Analyze ROI.** In other words, now that you've calculated your potential reimbursement and projected income, compare it to the up-front costs and support costs. This is rather basic, but you want your projected income to be more than your costs. What's your break-even point? How long will it take to get there? Is it worth the time, energy and value to your practice? ROI is Return on Investment.

> *"Now that you've calculated your potential reimbursement and projected income, compare it to the up-front costs and support costs. This is rather basic, but you want your projected income to be more than your costs."*

7. **Are there any contractual roadblocks?** If you've decided an ancillary business makes sense, take a look at potential problems. For instance, if you're offering the ancillary service in a leased space, review the lease agreement to see if there are any restrictions on how you can use that space. Leased space from a hospital or on a health care campus often has usage restrictions. Check with your malpractice insurance carrier to make sure your existing policy will cover the ancillary service or whether a rider is necessary or available (and factor in how much it will cost).

8. **Learn about the Stark Law.** If you decide to provide ancillary services, you should become familiar with the Stark Law, which is a provision of the Omnibus Budget Reconciliation Act of 1989 that was written by Congressman Pete Stark, that barred self-referrals for clinical lab services under Medicare. Within the ban against self-referrals were a myriad of exceptions to accommodate legitimate business relationships. The provisions were expanded in 1993, and again in 1994 and 1995. Essentially, the various Stark Laws and amendments prohibit physicians from referring patients for specific "designated health services" to a business entity and/or service that the physician has a financial relationship with if those services are paid for entirely or partially by Medicare or Medicaid—unless a Stark Law exception applies.

Although originally linked to physician office laboratories, it includes many other services, including x-ray, MRI, CT, PET, nuclear camera imaging, physical therapy, occupational therapy and outpatient prescription drugs. One of the exceptions is called the "in-office ancillary services" exception. The gist of this is that the Stark Law and its various amendments can complicate your life, so not only should you educate yourself about it, but consult with a practice management professional or attorney with experience in dealing with Stark Law prohibitions.

9. **Learn about the Antikickback Statute.** This is philosophically and legally similar to the Stark Laws. It was an amendment of the Medicare and Medicaid Patient Protection Act of 1987, and although it is fairly complex, it prohibits physicians from knowingly and willingly soliciting or receiving any remuneration, "including any kickback, bribe

or rebate (directly or indirectly, overtly or covertly, in cash or in kind—(A) in return for referring an individual to a person for the furnishing or arranging for the furnishing of any item or service for which payment may be made in whole or in part under [Medicare] or a State health care program."

There are other provisions, but perhaps the most important thing you need to keep in mind is that violating this statute is a felony which can result in a fine of $25,000 or 5 years in prison, or both. Again, consult with a practice management professional or attorney who has experience with this.

10. **Evaluate your plan under Medicare rules.** As if the Stark Laws and the Antikickback Statute weren't complicated enough, any physician who routinely deals with Medicare understands how many rules and regulations are involved. This goes double for any ancillary services you might offer, especially in the areas of rules over who can bill and collect for a particular service. For example, a physician goes to an outside radiologist to provide interpretations for the ancillary service, but the physician's practice bills and collects a global fee; that global fee includes the technical component and the professional component, which was provided by the radiologist. That can get complicated in a hurry.

Ancillary services can improve patient care, which is what it should ultimately be all about. It can also increase a physician's revenue. It can also double, triple or quadruple the work and hassle, if you don't plan carefully and explore what the many pros and cons of the individual service might be.

> **Action Step:** List 1 new service that your practice will provide within the next 12 months and cite your plan for implementation. Do this exercise on an annual basis.

ESSENTIAL #20:

In-office Dispensing

Should you become a product retailer?

One way to increase revenue and potentially make life more convenient for your patients is through in-office dispensing. That is to say, selling products in your office to patients. These products are related to your specialty of care, typically, and can range from moisturizers, over-the-counter medications and orthotics to dental floss, toothbrushes and contact lens cases.

There is a tendency for many physicians to recoil at the thought of offering products for sale in their offices, perhaps feeling there is a conflict between their professionalism and hawking products. This isn't a conflict that needs to exist, and it is our experience that patients do not find the sale of products in their physicians' offices to be in any way unprofessional, as long as the selling is low-key and relevant to their medical needs.

In fact, many patients appreciate the convenience. We have found 7 benefits to in-office dispensing:

1. *Improved patient satisfaction.* The products sold are of professional quality and patients appreciate the convenience of one-stop shopping.
2. *Increased patient compliance.* Since the product is right there in the office, and because the physician and/or staff can explain how to properly use the product, patients are more likely to purchase the right product and use it correctly.
3. *Complete patient care.* We have found that in-office dispensing makes patients feel as if we are providing more complete patient care, that we're not just prescribing a product or treatment, but making it readily available to them.
4. *Extra revenue.* The key here is to make it an ethical source of revenue, to make sure the products are ones you believe in and that will be of value to your patients. If patients are unhappy with the products you sell or find they don't trust the products you sell them, that can result in a loss of trust in you. But if you believe in the products and market them carefully, in-office dispensing can be a significant source of ancillary revenue for your practice and staff.
5. *Profit sharing.* More revenue for the practice can and should filter down to more benefits for your staff, particularly as they will be instrumental in any in-office sales. Share the wealth, create a profit-sharing plan and discover how well this can increase your staff's job satisfaction.
6. *More patient contact.* Patients often return to your office between visits to stock up on products.
7. *Increased patient referrals.* Current patients will often discuss their satisfaction with a product with friends and family and suggest they stop by the office (rather than the local Wal-Mart) to get the product.

One of the key things is the most simple of economic principles: The law of supply and demand. The patient is in need of a product (often recommended by you, the physician) and, instead of sending them outside of your office to get it, you supply it there.

In a November 2001 article in *Medical Economics*, it was reported that patients are willing to pay more—significantly more—out-of-pocket for prescriptions provided in the office just to avoid waiting in line at the pharmacy. Convenience is king.

How to begin?

First, spend a month keeping track of the patients that you send out of your office to buy a product or services from somewhere else. Write it down. Is it a prescription? An over-the-counter medication? Lotion? An orthotic? Special bandages or disinfectants? Eye drops?

Second, analyze that list to see what you could bring into your office. The important thing isn't to jump into it, but to carefully consider what you could sell in-office effectively. Does the product require refrigeration before sale? Special licensing? Bulk storage? Those could be real drawbacks.

Third, test the products yourself. As mentioned earlier, you have to be a believer in the products you're recommending and selling. It reflects on you as a physician if you recommend a product to a patient, but it can come crashing down on your head if you sell it in your office and patients have negative experiences with the products. Start with products you're already recommending. Visit your local pharmacy or retailer and explore the options.

> *"In a November 2001 article in* **Medical Economics,** *it was reported that patients are willing to pay more—significantly more— out-of-pocket for prescriptions provided in the office just to avoid waiting in line at the pharmacy."*

Fourth, look at the products for sale in your specialty's trade journals and magazines. Many of those products will work well in your practice and are easily stocked in-office. Many of those products are not widely available, which makes them an even better fit for you to sell.

Fifth, decide a price point. Sell at cost or add a profit margin? If you decide to sell at cost, remember to factor in the cost of shipping. Experiment with the price point and see how patients respond. But remember, although you want to increase revenue, you're also trying to make life more convenient for your patients.

Sixth, seriously think about how you will display and store items you plan to sell. They need to fit your office décor and not take up too much room. You also need storage for the items you carry. Suppliers offer Plexiglas display cases, which are convenient and still look professional. They're typically not very expensive.

How to approach sales?

Most practices that successfully perform in-house dispensing use what is called "passive marketing." In this technique, patients are not told they need to purchase a product.

Instead, the physician might say, "Ms. Jackson, you really need to use a skin moisturizer twice a day." Often, patients will ask for a recommendation, which gives the physician the opportunity to indicate what they offer as well as other products available on the market. Some offices use binders that contain their sales items for the patient to peruse.

We also recommend placing a sign in your reception room indicating that your office carries several products, perhaps with a note indicating that you have surveyed your patients and found that they appreciate the convenience.

Your staff should also be trained in this approach to "nonselling." Don't push a product, but demonstrate with it, and also indicate a similar product can be found in the local pharmacy, but it is available in your office if the patient would like to buy it now.

A collage of available products is a nice touch. Also, remind patients they can stop in to buy products any time they wish. During follow-up visits, ask patients if they are using the products, if they are using them as directed, and if they have run out or are running low.

Most importantly, make it clear that the patient visit isn't about selling them products, but simply a component of their treatment plan. Extend a full return policy for any reason at any time—physician first, retailers second.

In our experience, the initial investment runs between $3,000 and $5,000, but many practices create additional revenue ranging from $25,000–$100,000 through in-office dispensing.

There are a number of common questions we encounter:

Can physicians legally dispense prescription pharmaceuticals from their offices?

Yes, to their own patients. At this time, there are only 4 states that have some restrictions: New York, Montana, Texas and Massachusetts.

Will I need extra staff?

No. Existing staff can be trained and may benefit from an incentive program. It can be not only a great profit center, but a morale booster for staff.

Who can dispense medications or products in the office?

Most states allow an employee working under the direction and supervision of the licensed physician to dispense prescription medications or items. Some states require the physician, registered nurse, nurse practitioner or physician assistant to do the dispensing. Check your state laws.

Are items we dispense subject to sales tax?

Some are. Not all are. Your local accountant should be able to assist you on this.

> **Action Step:** List 3 products that you can immediately begin to dispense in your office. List how you plan to train your office team in presenting these products to your patients and develop treatment protocols for their use. Integrate 2–3 new products every 6 months with the same plan.

The Art Of Patient Communication And Compliance

Getting your patients to say "yes."
Presenting your treatment plan and getting patients to follow it.

Patient compliance is completely linked to a physician's communication skills. Fundamentally, we feel that there needs to be a shift away from being a "doctor" and a shift toward being a "caregiver." A caregiver carries less baggage than physician and the word by itself suggests the patient's best interests are at heart. In other words, a caregiver persuades a patient to do what is best for the patient; they get them to comply.

A noncompliant patient is the bane of health care and several studies suggest that noncompliance costs the US health care system more than $100 billion annually. Much of that noncompliance is the fault of physicians and poor communication skills.

We present 6 rules for improving caregiver-patient communication, which can lead to higher levels of patient compliance.

1. *Active listening.* It's not enough to simply listen to a patient's words. You need to learn to listen to the patient's emotions that those words convey. There's an important word to describe this: Empathy. By connecting with the patient emotionally, you reflect back their emotions, which is a powerful bridge to credibility and trustworthiness, the building blocks of persuasion.

2. *Decisiveness.* Not only does the physician need to *be* decisive, the physician needs to communicate in a decisive manner. Physicians often use words or phrases such as "I think" and "maybe," but those can instill doubt and even confuse patients. Alternately, words such as "critical" and "essential" are perceived as decisive and add weight to the physician's message.

   We recommend that you even prepare scripts for your most common presentations. Craft those scripts so they flow and sound natural, but also to eliminate any vague or wishy-washy sounding language. An example:

   Poor: *"I think you might need an antibiotic for this infection."*

   Good: *"It's essential that we get you on an antibiotic so you can get well faster."*

   Part of the strategy is to incorporate what the patient wants and needs into your delivery. What does the patient want? To feel better sooner.

> *"Part of the strategy is to incorporate what the patient wants and needs into your delivery. What does the patient want? To feel better sooner."*

3. *Association.* It's important when you are crafting your scripts that you make the language accessible to the patient. Patients are often confused by medical language, but won't necessarily express that confusion to you out of embarrassment or for fear of appearing stupid. One way to improve your communication with patients is to associate medical terminology with more common language. An example:

    Poor: *"I think you need an orthotic for your heel pain."*

    Good: *"In order to help you resolve your pain, it's essential that I get you into an orthotic. Orthotics are removable inserts made by an impression of your feet. They help control the mechanical weakness in your feet, much like eyeglasses control weakness of the eyes."*

4. *Contrast.* Not only explain the value of a proposed treatment plan, but describe what could happen if the patient doesn't comply. An example:

    Poor: *"I think you need an antibiotic to clear up this earache."*

    Good: *"It's critical that we clear up this earache quickly, using an antibiotic so it doesn't spread into a full-fledged sinus infection. And it's important that you complete the prescription and take all of the medications, not just until you feel better. If you quit too early, the infection may come back tougher than ever and run the risk of being resistant to antibiotics."*

5. *The Two-by-Four Rule.* By any other name this is: You never get a second chance to make a first impression. Basically, research tells us that the impression you make on someone in the first 2 seconds upon meeting them takes 4 minutes to change. So when, as a physician, you enter the examining room, your immediate impression on the patient will have a lasting effect on your credibility and trustworthiness. Dress appropriately, professionally and neatly. Make eye contact and maintain good posture. Avoid condescending language. Be friendly. Smile!

6. *UPOD.* An excellent acronym that stands for: Under-Promise and Over-Deliver. Although we recommend you be decisive in your language and avoid waffling, any physician knows that there are no 100% guarantees in medicine. Be careful of words such as "always" and "never." Use works such as "likely" to avoid making promises or guarantees.

In addition, we feel there are nuances you can bring to your patient-physician communications, or perhaps this is a good time to emphasize *patient-caregiver* communications. There is great value in the power of touch. That can begin with a handshake and, in many forms of physician-patient interactions, there are reasons to appropriately touch a patient. Studies show that, for instance, taking a patient's foot or hand in both hands conveys compassion.

Stay away from yes-and-no questions. Start your interaction with a question related to the patient's overall health and well-being, such as "How have you been?" This type of open question can, unfortunately, lead you offtrack if you have a chatty patient, so you need to be able to focus the conversation to the particular problem the patient comes in for. So, another opening gambit might be, "So, what brings you here today?" Be careful about interrupting the patient early in the encounter, because this will make the patient feel rushed.

Patients already assume you provide quality medical care. What gives you a competitive edge are your people skills. Mary Kay Ash, the founder of Mary Kay Cosmetics, claimed that the secret of her success was to make people feel important. In our medical practices, the goal isn't just to provide care, but to make all our patients feel special, that they are our top priority. To that end, the physician needs to not just aim for a satisfied patient, but a "Wow" experience. This starts from their very first contact with your staff in the form of the telephone call or when the patient walks through the door.

> *"In our medical practices, the goal isn't just to provide care,*
> *but to make all our patients feel special, that they are our top priority.*
> *To that end, the physician needs to not just aim for a*
> *satisfied patient, but a 'Wow' experience."*

We believe the phone should be answered in fewer than 3 rings. Whoever answers the phone provides their name in the greeting and, if it is necessary to put the patient on hold, asks for their permission to do so. Thank them for holding and, at the end of the conversation, make sure your staff asks if the patients have any questions or need anything else. Your staff should be encouraged or trained to make eye contact with patients and smile. If you're running behind, patients should be informed of the wait.

Be aware of and attentive to The Doorknob Moment. The Doorknob Moment involves this scenario: The physician stands up to end the patient visit, but before standing up asks if the patient has anything else they want to discuss. The patient says, "No." The physician stands up to leave, puts his or her hand on the doorknob, and the patient says, "There is one thing . . ."

Often, the thing the patient really has on her mind is the very thing she brings up at the last minute. (Not always, but often). Often, it's a major issue. Part of this phenomenon may be tied to the results of a study conducted in the 1980s that found doctors interrupt patients on an average of just 18 seconds into a routine office visit, making patients feel rushed.

One technique to decrease The Doorknob Moment is to provide a patient with a 3x5 index card and a pen or pencil when they arrive. Have your staff tell them to write down any questions they may have for the physician that day.

Another way to avoid this is to actively listen and to simply ask, "Is there anything else I can help you with today?"

Action Step: Create effective scripts for your 5 most frequent patient dialogues, for both the front office and the clinical team. Practice the scripts regularly at special office meetings. Add 5 new scripts monthly until all are completed.

Five Steps To Plugging Revenue Leakage

Collecting co-pays, evaluating financials regularly,
creating benchmarks and asking for your money.
Don't assume because it's small you can ignore it.

Revenue leakage is a simple concept. Think of your house. Do you have a sink that drips? A window that lets in drafts?

A medical practice can be just like that—a little leak here, a little leak there. Are you collecting all your co-pays? Are any accounts overdue? They may seem minor, but they add up, or they go on too long and you stop thinking about them . . . until you realize you're losing a lot of money.

Many physicians make the crucial mistake of assuming everything is coming along just fine. Of course, it's possible that everything *is* coming along just fine. It's also possible the wheels are about to fall off your practice because you haven't bothered to check that the lug nuts are tight. Although we will offer 5 steps to plug any revenue leakage, a prelist step is to Never Assume.

> *"Many physicians make the crucial mistake of assuming everything*
> *is coming along just fine. Of course, it's possible that everything is*
> *coming along just fine. It's also possible the wheels are about to fall*
> *off your practice because you haven't bothered to check that the lug*
> *nuts are tight. Although we will offer 5 steps to plug any*
> *revenue leakage, a prelist step is to Never Assume."*

You want to empower your staff to work on accounts receivable and to handle billing issues. The problem is that physicians then lose track of what's actually going on in their practice's business operations. You don't have to take over those responsibilities, but staying on top of money matters is important.

- Do you meet regularly with your staff to review reports?
- Do you have financial benchmarks?
- Do you compare what's happening this year compared to what happened last year?
- Do you know what's normal in other specialties?
- Do you audit charts?
- Do you evaluate 10 charts a month to see if they're entered properly?

We also suggest you periodically hire a professional billing service (if you do your own billing) to spend a day auditing your charts and receivables.

Five other ways to plug revenue leakage are:

1. *Ask for your money.* Very few people are comfortable asking for money, even when it's owed. Medical people, in particular, seem to have problems collecting money. Maybe it has something to do with the caregiver mentality. Nonetheless, unless you're planning on operating a nonprofit or charity, people have bills to pay. Don't be shy. If a patient owes you a co-pay, ask for it. We recommend you collect it up front as much as possible. Put procedures in place that makes it as easy as possible to collect your money—accept cash, checks and credit cards. There are exceptions, of course, but working hard to make sure no one leaves the office without paying their co-pay or their bill will go a long way toward keeping your ship from springing a leak.

2. *Lay out estimated expenses.* When you meet with a patient prior to an expensive procedure, particularly surgery or something complicated, create a financial agreement ahead of time so the patient knows how much the procedure will cost. Put it in writing and get the patient to agree to it by signing it. Both the patient and your practice get a copy. It's especially good to have this in writing, because patients are often nervous and distracted when discussing major medical procedures. Having it in writing allows them to review it at home when they can concentrate on it.

3. *Audit your computer systems.* There is a tendency to blindly trust computer systems, particularly those that handle billing. Often, they're remarkably reliable, but they also create a false security of security—do you really know what the computer system is doing? Sometimes there are features on practice management software that can cause inadvertent problems. For example, one piece of office management software required that after you save your transaction, you hit Print Claim. The claim then is sent electronically. But if you don't hit Print Claim, it doesn't get sent and it shows up as an outstanding balance, even though the insurance company never received it. This goes back to Never Assume. Although you may not be eager to learn the ins and outs of your practice management software, it's important that you understand what its capabilities and limitations are, and to double-check regularly to make sure it's doing what you think it's doing.

4. *Offer appropriate services.* It's surprising to us how many physicians don't offer complete services that could bring in additional revenue. This isn't to suggest that you offer services that are medically inappropriate, but rather that if a patient comes in with a specific ailment, it may be an opportunity to offer a more thorough checkup that could result in more services and care, which not only results in better and more comprehensive care for the patient, but more revenue for the physician. It's possible there may be preventive measures you could address in dealing with a specific ailment. These extras are perfectly good medicine and insurance will pay for them.

5. *Nag the insurers.* As most physicians will attest, it's rare to file an insurance claim and get exactly what you're supposed to. Regularly update your contracts with insurers, go through your price lists and send them to insurance companies. Occasionally, insurance carriers change their reimbursement and, even less occasionally, they increase their reimbursements, but it happens often enough to make it worth evaluating.

Appealing claims can be a good idea as well. Errors occur on the insurance company side as well and it might turn out that they do owe you more money, anywhere from $80–$500. This applies to Medicare as well, and we recommend that you get to know your state Medicare liaison and join your state's specialty medical association so you can tap into their resources in dealing with insurers.

All of these steps can help you prevent slow money leakage. Aside from embezzlement, however, the worst cause of revenue leakage is losing patients. Losing patients is revenue leakage. An unsatisfied patient is revenue leakage. Have happy, satisfied patients and you've plugged a significant source of revenue leakage in your practice.

> **Action Step:** List 2 collection strategies for your front office team and also your billing team that you will employ this year to boost your revenue.

Time Management

Get off the gerbil wheel and control your life and practice.

A re you busy? Of course you are. Not only are you a physician, but you're running a business. For years, we've run full-time practices as well as acted as medical practice management consultants and speakers. Over the years, we've learned a few things—hopefully—about managing our time. Here are 13 tips we've found helpful.

1. **Master Schedule.** Having 1 schedule for the practice that indicates your schedule, the employees' schedules, patients' schedules and everything else on it helps significantly. Everyone on staff needs to feed into the master schedule so that all relevant professional activities, as well as special occasions (birthdays, holidays, etc) are available at a glance. Professional activities can include normal office hours, nursing home visits, surgical appointments, house calls, teaching and workshop dates, conferences and educational seminars. But it's not enough to just make the schedule—you have to look at it. Make sure you look at the next day's schedule prior to the end of your work day so you won't be surprised by anything on the schedule. *Oops! I'm giving a talk tomorrow and I haven't made the PowerPoint slides yet!*

2. **Ask For Help.** If you're really having problems being organized, discuss it with your staff. Set up a mutually convenient time when you won't be interrupted (like a Saturday morning, perhaps) and brainstorm about how to avoid wasting time and increasing efficiency.

3. **Analyze Appointment Patterns.** This can be surprisingly effective. Are there some patients that you know suck up your time? Are there certain types of exams that require more time (like physicals)? What are your busiest days? What are your slowest days? Perhaps there are certain days when certain types of appointments would be better (eg, scheduling physicals for Fridays, if they're your slowest days). If you're traveling between practice locations, are you scheduling travel time? Identify problem areas and adjust your scheduling patterns accordingly.

4. **Block Out Times.** Sometimes our days seem horribly fragmented, going from 1 type of task to another to another. This is terribly inefficient and can be energy draining as well. Increase efficiency by scheduling blocks of time for things that are similar—surgical assistance or minor office procedures, or physicals all on 1 day, or nursing home visits all scheduled at once, or 1 day that is devoted to immunizations or allergy shots.

5. **Interrupt The Interruptions.** How much time do you spend getting interrupted? Hundreds of times a day? Are you interrupted by your staff? Interrupted by patients? By sales people? By family and friends? (By email, Facebook, Twitter and dozens of other so-called social media?) This happens to everybody, but it can be a huge time

sink. Patients need to make appointments, and so do pharmaceutical reps and, yes, even family members. If necessary, schedule time in for interruptions and appointments when you deal with non–patient-related business.

6. **Multitask.** Most physicians do this, but take a harder look at how and when you're doing it. Can you keep multiple examining rooms running simultaneously? Are all your examining rooms properly stocked so everything you need is in every room? Are they all organized appropriately and easy to find?

7. **Dictation Or A Scribe.** There are a number of charting possibilities, thanks to current technology. Some physicians prefer to write their own charts. Others dictate and pay someone to type them up. Others hire scribes, who follow you around from room to room and take notes. There is quite a bit of practice management software that allows you to program in certain levels of regular responses into your notes, which can save an enormous amount of time. Although some cost more than others, they often pay for themselves quickly through efficiency.

8. **Stay Ahead Of The Paperwork.** Although everybody's work style varies, in general, it's far more efficient to stay ahead of your paperwork by working on it daily rather than letting it pile up until you can't find your desk beneath all the dead tree stuff. One recommendation is to touch paper only once—file it, shred it or give it to someone to do something about it. Don't touch it to move it to another pile when you'll get around to it later. Also, when you work out your billing fees, take into consideration the time you need to spend finishing paperwork not covered by insurers.

9. **Schedule An Extra Day.** If you're traveling, whether on business or on vacation, consider scheduling an extra day in the office to catch up on paperwork and miscellaneous catch-up before seeing patients. There's nothing worse than coming back from a vacation and immediately feeling overwhelmed and behind.

10. **Prepare Advice Sheets.** If you regularly give out the same advice to patients for specific illnesses, prepare pamphlets or handouts that you can give to the patients. Patients typically glaze over at extensive verbal directions, but preprinted materials, particularly with relevant areas highlighted or circled, can give the patient more time to go over them and save you the time of explaining the same thing 50 times a week.

11. **Get Away.** One thing about self-employment—it can take over your life. And the Internet, smartphones, laptop computers and iPads have made it all too easy to take your work with you. Try to disconnect from work. When you're home, you're home; when you're on vacation, you're on vacation. Even if you have to schedule time away, do it. Not only will this help you be more efficient when you are at work, it'll help keep burnout at bay.

12. **Study Your Workflow.** Every process, whether it's building a car or seeing patients, becomes engrained: *"We've always done it this way!"* The entire LEAN and Six-Sigma analysis in manufacturing came about because there are numerous inefficiencies built into most systems and people don't want to change and don't realize things might be

faster and easier a different way. Several years ago, a major hospital brought in a LEAN expert to see if he could increase efficiency on 1 of the patient floors. The first thing he did was have the nurses wear pedometers. He found rather quickly that nurses on the patient floor were walking an average of 5 miles a day *just because the drug cabinet was located on a different hallway!* It was an easy fix and dramatically increased efficiency. Study what's going on in your own practice. Are there things you do that don't make sense or inadvertently waste time? Change them!

Our **13th** recommendation requires some more time to discuss. It is: **Delegate.** We define delegation as "the art of assigning responsibility and authority to key staff of an organization in order to improve productivity." We have typically found that there are 5 common reasons that physicians don't delegate. They are:

1. You haven't taken the time to really look at what you do and how you do it, so you're not sure what you could delegate successfully.
2. You're a micromanager and think you need to do everything yourself. Yes, control freak, you!
3. You don't have confidence (trust) in your staff.
4. You like the stress of doing it yourself.
5. You might feel guilty about giving work to other people in order to free up time for yourself.

Because delegation is something of a skill in itself, or perhaps it's even an art, we have come up with 8 considerations to assist in making you a better delegator.

1. *Analyze everything you do.* Make lists of big projects and break down the small details. Those can include phone calls, applications and writing notes. Make the list very detailed. Then, check off the ones that can be done by someone else or that you would like to get rid of. Then, underline the ones which you think only you can do or those that you want to keep for yourself.
2. *Who can do the ones you checked off?* Now that you have a list of things you can delegate or want to delegate, identify the person on your staff that you think would be best suited to do it. You need to determine if this person is not only capable of performing these tasks, but whether he or she has the time to do it. This may require you to analyze what skills are required to perform these tasks. It's important that you either match up the person with the appropriate skills to do the job, or the person who is most willing and able to learn how to do it.
3. *Request vs order.* Not all staff members are necessarily eager to take on a new job. Sometimes it's because they feel they're already too busy (and they might be), or there's something about the task they don't like. They may also be concerned that the task is beyond them and they might screw it up; if that's the case, some encouragement on your part is in order. You want to empower your employees whenever possible. So, request that the person take on this task or ask them if they would be interested in it. Use respect and show your appreciation.

4. *Communicate.* Like most areas of being a physician or managing people, communication is key. You need to have a clear picture of what you want achieved when you delegate a task and then need to communicate that to the person you're delegating it to. Don't assume the person you're asking to do something understands why you're asking them or exactly why you want the task done. Also, to further empower an employee, if it isn't essential that the task be performed in a precise way, allow them the chance to use their initiative and creativity to approach the project differently than you would. This can result is spectacular new ways of accomplishing things.

5. *Break it down.* If a task is complicated, break it down into a step-by-step action plan.

6. *Why.* As mentioned in #4, include why you want the task performed, as well as why you're asking them to do it. People function better when they understand the motivation for doing something. You also need to make it clear that you're asking them to do it because they're capable of it and you trust them to do it, not that you're assigning them extra work as punishment or because you think they're not busy enough.

7. *Equilibrate the oversight.* Most people don't like having a supervisor breathing down their neck. Some people can barely function with a micromanager hovering and others require some line-of-sight supervision. Adjust your level of oversight based on the skill levels and experience of the person you're delegating to, and to the type of task you're delegating. With time, an empowered employee won't require much supervision.

8. *Provide feedback.* Most people do not do things perfectly the first time. Feedback is required and it's your job to provide appropriate feedback when you delegate tasks to people. Tell them what they did well and tell them what they need to improve on. Again, if you have negative feedback to provide, placing it into a context of why the job wasn't up to standards gives the employee an understanding, not only of what they need to do, but why they need to do it in a specific way. And remember, positive feedback is important. If you only provide feedback when you're unhappy with the way things are going, you won't get the results you're hoping for.

And 1 final tip: **Prioritize.** None of us can accomplish everything, and trying to is a surefire way to burn out early and fast. Decide what's most important and concentrate on accomplishing those things. The less important things can be delegated or can wait for time to open up.

> **Action Step:** Create an activity log to assess how you spend your time over a 14-day period. List 3 things over a 1-month period that you can do in order to optimize your time. Then, 1 month later, do the same exercise. Keep a daily log of 1 thing you do for yourself that is important to you. It can be simple.

Bringing On An Associate
Or Additional Associates

How to bring on an associate or partner,
and what to consider before you do.

There may come a time when you decide you want a partner or associate. The reasons for this may vary: You're very busy and want to take more time for yourself and your family; the volume of your practice has grown to such a degree that you need someone to help with it; you're considering retirement soon enough that you're thinking about eventually selling the practice. All of those are good reasons to bring in an associate or partner and should each be evaluated independently and thoroughly before making the decision, which is a major one.

Before bringing in a partner or associate, you need to remember that this is very similar to hiring an employee, only the stakes are even higher. You also need to know what your goals are by bringing in another physician. Do you want more time off? Are you interested in increasing volume or diversifying your procedural capabilities? What do you hope to achieve?

Here are some questions we recommend you ask yourself before beginning the process.

- What do you hope to achieve?
- What sort of credentials should a partner or associate have to help you achieve that goal?
- If your goal is to increase the overall patient visit volume, how will this affect the practice's total expenses?
- How many patients does the practice need to see (ie, what is the patient volume level that you will need for your practice's optimal profit margin)?
- Is your office infrastructure capable of handling the additional patients? And that infrastructure can apply to office, examining rooms and reception rooms, as well as office staff.
- Is your office's location (ie, community) conducive to your practice's growth?
- Are you ready to manage another physician?
- Are you willing to give up some of the control and decision making in your practice?

Once you've given some thought to those questions, you can start thinking about where to find a partner or associate. It's possible you'll have someone in mind from your interactions with colleagues in your area, or people you've worked with or interacted with at conferences. Otherwise, you need to open it up through outside resources, like journals in your specialty or online resources. There are also recruiting firms specializing in physician practices and specialties that can help you find a qualified candidate.

There are some things to consider besides the potential partner's technical qualifications. Personality, of course, is a major factor. You want to get along well with your partner. But at least as important is making sure that the prospective associate understands what your goals are. If you, as the senior partner, plan to travel or be out of the office more, then the associate needs to understand up front that 1 of the reasons you're hiring him or her is so you can get out of the office. If it's to increase patient volume, they need to understand that as well.

> *"There are some things to consider besides the potential partner's technical qualifications. Personality, of course, is a major factor. You want to get along well with your partner. But at least as important is making sure that the prospective associate understands what your goals are."*

Another factor has to do with the corporate culture your practice has. That includes the personality and philosophy of your practice and office staff. Sometimes you need to meet the candidate in a social setting with your staff as well as in a more traditional, interview-type venue. Considerations are, do you and the candidate have the same philosophy regarding patient care, can the candidate meet your goals and are they willing to? Also, is the candidate comfortable living and working in the community where your practice is located?

Now that you have a person in mind for the partnership or associateship, you need to decide—both of you, quite likely—on how compensation will be designed. There are typically 3 methods of associate compensation:

- Pure salary
- Pure percentage of production based on percentage of income
- Salary plus incentive

Each method has risks for either you or the associate. A *pure salary strategy* for the associate puts all the risk on you. Will the associate generate enough income to warrant the compensation?

In a pure percentage of production strategy, the associate is taking more of the risk. He or she can't predict if patient volume will shift or increase. Also, from your point of view, this requires that you seek legal advice to make sure you don't violate any antikickback laws.

The most common method is a *base salary plus an incentive*, which shares the risk between the senior partner (you) and the associate. The associate is paid a nominal base salary and receives a bonus after a specific preset level of income is generated. Our recommendation is that the income threshold be approximately 3 times the associate's base salary. For example, if you decide the base salary is $50,000 annually, the associate is rewarded a bonus starting when they have generated $150,000 of practice income.

Typically, a percentage of each dollar made above that threshold payment is awarded, usually 15%–25%. So, once the associate brings in $150,000 of revenue to the practice, they start earning 15–25 cents on every dollar they bring in. This bonus can be calculated and paid out monthly or quarterly. The advantages of this system are that it gives the associate continual feedback as well as incentives and active participation in the practice's financial health.

Other factors other than salary and bonuses to be negotiated are:

- Vacations
- Malpractice insurance
- Health insurance
- Disability insurance
- CME allowances
- Dues and subscriptions
- Auto/gas allowances
- Fees for licenses and boards, managed care privileges and hospital applications

Naturally, the days of handshake deals are long gone, if they ever existed. An associate must sign a contract of employment. It protects both of you. There are also many state and federal regulations requiring written employment agreements. It should be designed by both parties and prepared by an attorney familiar with medical practice agreements. The agreement should include:

- Employment duties and performance
- Terms of employment
- Compensation package, including base pay and incentives
- Responsibilities regarding maintenance of office facilities
- Death/disability/worker's compensation
- Malpractice insurance
- Issues pertaining to ownership of medical records
- Covenant not to compete/not to solicit
- Termination clauses

You may also include language regarding interactions with staff and staff hiring and firing. The associate's responsibilities and expected duties should be made clear and be reasonably detailed. Should covenants be broken, liquidated damages can be discussed in the contract, as well as details of termination clauses. An attorney can help lay out what is usual in your state.

Once an associate is brought on, it's up to you to help that partner integrate into your practice. You will need to introduce the new associate to patients as well as local physicians, and do a sales job detailing your new associate's credentials and capabilities.

Sit down with the associate to go over practice protocols, which should be reviewed and mutually agreed upon. It's important that you and your associate present a single and consistent style and image to patients, as much as possible. The office staff needs to be educated on the associate's role and how they should present the associate's business and relationship to patients.

Although it is your responsibility to provide clear and consistent feedback to the new associate, you are also colleagues. Let the associate participate in management decisions and listen to their feedback. The associate has a stake in the success of the practice and brings a set of fresh eyes and perspective to the practice. Keep an open-book policy in terms of the practice's finances, which will build a sense of trust and empower the associate.

> **Action Step:** List what factors in your practice and personal life could initiate consideration of an associate. Knowing your current situation, develop a timeframe for those factors.

Non-medical Malpractice Insurance Coverage

Malpractice insurance is a given, but what other types of insurance should your practice have?

With very few exceptions, physicians will have medical malpractice insurance. And if you're running a practice with employees (or even if you're not), you're probably dealing with health insurance for yourself and your employees. However, as small business owners, there are several other types of insurance you need that will protect you and your practice. There are 7 categories:

- Comprehensive general liability
- Property coverage
- Business income interruption
- Workers' compensation
- Automobile
- Disability
- Employment-related practices

We'll cover them one at a time.

COMPREHENSIVE GENERAL LIABILITY INSURANCE

This type of insurance protects you from things that might happen to people on your practice's property. Typically, this refers to things like slip-and-fall accidents. They are not related to the actual care of the patient.

PROPERTY COVERAGE INSURANCE

If you rent or own the building your practice is in, you're going to need some sort of property coverage. This covers things like fire- and weather-related damage. There is also coverage for specific types of professional property. For instance, there is coverage that deals with the loss of patient records, losses of medicines caused by temperature changes or for coverage for accounts receivable. There's even coverage for damage or vandalism that occurs to your practice's signage.

BUSINESS INCOME INTERRUPTION INSURANCE

Like the name indicates, business income interruption insurance covers loss of income if, for some reason, you can't earn income. For instance, if your practice burns down, property coverage should cover the cost of rebuilding the building. However, it won't cover the loss of income during the period the building is being rebuilt. Business income insurance does. If an ice storm knocks out the power for a week (or a hurricane or flood), business income interruption insurance provides the coverage. This is a type of insurance that many people are unaware of, but it can make a huge difference if something happens to your practice that prevents you from operating for a period of time.

WORKERS' COMPENSATION

This is designed to cover your employees if they should become injured while working.

AUTOMOBILE INSURANCE

Although you'll need car insurance for yourself personally, if you use your vehicle to travel between practice locations, it's important that you have insurance that covers this. In particular, if you are traveling from office location to office location and should get in an accident, the other person involved might sue. The result of that lawsuit may be to go after other assets, such as those involved with your practice, so having automobile insurance that covers for that contingency is worthwhile.

DISABILITY INSURANCE

There are 2 different categories of disability insurance: Personal disability insurance and overhead disability insurance. Although the definitions may differ a bit from insurance company to insurance company, most major insurance companies have what is called an "own-occupation" definition of disability. This is defined to mean that if you can't perform the specific duties of your occupation due to injury or illness, you will be considered disabled and can receive benefits.

This varies from medical practitioner to medical practitioner—a surgeon's disability might be different from a general practitioner's disability. Richard Reich, President of Intramark Insurance Services, Inc., in Los Angeles, describes it this way: "The best definition of his 'own-occupation' would allow him/her (the physician) to participate in another occupation and still receive disability benefits if it's deemed he or she still can't perform the duties of the occupation. The better types of coverage limit that to single medical specialties."

Insurers tend to take a long, hard look at the physician's financial background before granting this type of insurance, because they want to be able to pick a benefit rate that's appropriate for the physician's income level. With group disability insurance policies, it's typically 60%–66% of the physician's income. There are taxation differences between group and individual policies, which will vary from state to state and policy to policy.

Coverage for disability insurance typically is applicable to the age of 65, sometime 67. Some insurers will offer lifetime coverage. The cost is usually 1%–3% of your income.

Overhead disability insurance is slightly different. For instance, if a physician is injured and wants to keep the practice operating while injured, business overhead insurance keeps the doors open and the employees paid until the physician can return to work. Disability insurance covers personal expenses and income; overhead disability insurance covers the overhead of the business as well as the personal.

Additional factors to consider with disability insurance are *recovery benefit* or *residual benefit*. If a physician is injured and misses a period of work, then returns to practice but it takes time to build the practice back up again, the insurance pays for a percentage of lost income. Also, cost of living increases should be built into the policy; you also want to be able to increase your benefits without having to prove medical eligibility or take medical exams.

EMPLOYMENT-RELATED PRACTICES INSURANCE

Employment-related practices insurance covers lawsuits for things that might come up during the course of employment: Discrimination, harassment, wrongful termination, failure to hire.

When you look at this type of insurance, the first question that comes up is, "How much coverage do I need?" This becomes a strictly financial question, by and large. For instance, if you want $1 million in coverage, which might cost you $700 a year, or $2 million in coverage that will cost you $1,500 a year, it might make sense to go with the $1 million in coverage. If the difference between the two is only $100, for instance, from $700 to $800, then the $2 million coverage makes sense.

The second question involves how much your deductible should be. Another way of putting this is: If you get sued and are covered, how much of the claim do you want to pay yourself? Of course, when the deductible goes up, the premium goes down, and vice versa.

For both areas, take into consideration the cost of defense. As you pay your lawyer, you use up your insurance. Although many of these types of claims eventually get thrown out of court, the attorneys continue to get paid until they do.

There are also what are often considered "internal issues," which typically come down to definitions of a "wrongful act." The policies typically are written to indicate they will cover the physician for a "wrongful act." Then the policy very specifically defines a wrongful act.

For instance, a policy will say it will cover you from discrimination. Then it will define discrimination. Some policies will provide coverage for sexual harassment, others only for workplace harassment. But the definitions tend to be very clear and precise, forcing you to either choose numerous categories or hope that the language is broad enough to allow for broad coverage.

Typically, these types of coverage are relatively inexpensive compared to health insurance and medical malpractice insurance. However, if you have 6 or 7 of them, they add up. Many major insurers have combined insurance policies for small business owners. Still, each policy runs somewhere around $600–$1,000 each per year, which is going to run you somewhere around $4,000–$6,000. Balance that against your per-patient visit rate and you can start to calculate exactly how many patients you need to see just to pay your insurance bill. For example, if you have a $6,000 insurance bill and your per-patient visit rate is $100, then you need to see 60 patients just to pay for your non-medical malpractice insurance. You need to balance that with the knowledge that a fire or lawsuit could wipe out your entire practice permanently.

AN OUNCE OF PREVENTION . . .

Insurance coverage gives you protection after the fact. However, there are certain things you can do to minimize risk or to prevent accidents or lawsuits.

One thing is to put in a surveillance system. If someone slips or falls, or something is stolen, having security cameras inside and outside your practice can provide documentation of what actually happened. Surveillance cameras need to be located in such a way that everyone—patients included—can see them. There are some obvious locations that are not appropriate—examining rooms and bathrooms. Also, make sure that you don't inadvertently place a camera in a location that takes shots into a patient room if the patient leaves the door cracked a bit. But the parking lot and reception area are good locations for risk management.

> *"Consistency is required. Having a policy and not following it can make you just as liable as not having a policy."*

It's a good idea to run a background check on anyone you plan to hire. It can be a criminal background check, which is obvious; however, you can also run a financial background check, which can see if someone has a bad history of debt or if someone was fired or arrested for stealing things. Not finding out if someone has a criminal history and they are caught stealing makes you, as the employer, liable.

In cases of harassment lawsuits, office manuals need to clearly and prominently have language stating who the complainant can go to and what the procedures are for dealing with a variety of harassment types. Some states require this, and if they do and you don't have a written policy about it, you have little or no defense against a lawsuit. Also, document behavior. If there's an incident that occurs, whether it resulted in termination or not, you need to document what was done about it. If your office manual states the first step is a verbal warning, you need to document that a verbal warning was made and when. Consistency is required. Having a policy and not following it can make you just as liable as not having a policy.

Finally, make sure that the policies you do get cover what you think they cover. A good insurance agent will point out areas of vulnerability. However, you need to know what your coverage is. Stay informed.

> **Action Plan:** Review your medical malpractice policy to be sure you are covered appropriately in all areas and get an estimate from 1 other medical malpractice insurance company.

Thoughts On Office Design

Efficiency, storage and décor.

Whether you're building an office space from scratch or "building out" a leased space, a medical office has unique needs and problems to be addressed. It's a good time to point out that although you, as a physician, might have some idea of what you think you need in a practice space, an architect, designer or building contractor with experience designing medical spaces can provide insights that may never have occurred to you.

EFFICIENCY

Although this may seem a little obvious, a solo physician needs less space than a practice with multiple physicians. However, efficiency isn't isolated to either one—giving some thought to where things are and how the arrangement of rooms affects workflow can lead to an efficient workspace.

A few basics: Exam rooms should be, as much as possible, identical to each other. This means everything—tables, chairs, sink, instrument tray, storage space, tissue box, prescription pad—are in the exact same location. This not only leads to efficiency, it decreases stress, because you won't have to hunt for what you want or remind yourself where things are in each room.

There is another fact that needs to be balanced with efficiency. What is your office's "feel"? Many practitioners go with a fairly standard office setup, which can be quite bland while remaining professional. Both John and Hal have decorated their offices with things they are passionate about. In Hal's case, his entire practice has a "Wizard of Oz" theme, with a yellow brick road painted on the wall and a variety of Oz collectibles on display. John, too, chooses to have a motif, in his case, classic movies, with a variety of film posters decorating his walls.

> *"Others prefer a neutral style, which can be totally appropriate,*
> *as long as you don't become too clinical and cold. You want patients*
> *to feel comfortable and welcomed, but there's no reason to confuse*
> *them by making your practice look like a Chinese restaurant when*
> *they walk in the door . . . unless there's a good reason for that."*

Although that personal touch works for them, it may not work for all practices. A pediatrician may want something more child oriented, an OB/GYN possibly baby focused. Others prefer a neutral style, which can be totally appropriate, as long as you don't become too clinical and cold. You want patients to feel comfortable and welcomed, but there's no reason to confuse them by making your practice look like a Chinese restaurant when they walk in the door . . . unless there's a good reason for that.

PRIVACY

Of course, the examining rooms need to provide privacy for patients. What can sometimes cause problems are the layout of rooms as they relate to each other: The x-ray room to the exam room to the bathroom where urine samples may be collected. Patients don't want to parade from room to room down a lengthy hallway or around corners, so having the x-ray room and bathroom centrally located will help minimize traffic and patient exposure.

Some practices like to have a separate check-in and check-out area. One fairly easy way to do this is to have the check-in area in the reception area and the check-out area in the hallway just outside the reception area, with the staff area centrally located. This relieves bottlenecks at the front desk.

Many practices have a glass partition at the desk that can be closed off at either location. This is a fairly traditional aspect of physician's offices, even though some physicians believe an open space makes things feel more open and friendly. However, not being able to close off the office from where patients are waiting can be inconvenient for routine discussions between physician and staff, whether related to specific patients or not. The key, if you do go with the sliding glass window or door, is to make sure that it doesn't become a barrier. As soon as a patient enters the reception area, the door should be opened, even if it's just long enough to say, "Just one moment, please. We'll be right with you."

ALLOCATION OF SPACE

Space needs vary a great deal from practice specialty to practice specialty, as well as from single practices to group practices. A solo practitioner might make do with a minimum of 800 square feet, but that number increases significantly based on the technology used in the practice or types of ancillary services or in-office dispensing the practice offers. Having multiple physicians doesn't necessarily lead to an equal expansion; in other words, if a single practitioner utilizes 800 square feet, 3 practitioners can't necessarily get away with 2,400 square feet (800×3). Some space requirements are the same, but administrative space, patient reception areas and treatment areas increase exponentially.

A fairly standard calculation for determining the size of your reception area is to multiply the number of patients you expect to see during your busiest hour times 2.5 to account for "tag-along" relatives and friends. For instance, if you have 4 patients per hour, you get 10. You then subtract from that the number of exam rooms you have to get the number of chairs you will need (10–3=7). Finally, to determine square footage of the reception area, multiple that number of chairs by 20 square feet (7×20=140 square feet).

A standard figure for treatment rooms is a minimum of 8 feet by 8 feet. Depending on your local building codes, plumbing may be required in each treatment room and is highly recommended, anyway. Parking size is also often specified by local building codes.

And again, as said earlier, specialties and subspecialties have different requirements. Will your facility have surgical space? Will you have paper patient files, electronic health records or both? If you sell ancillary products, what kind will you sell? What kind of storage is required? What kind of display space? A laboratory often has specific space requirements and laboratory equipment can often take up a great deal of space, depending on the type and the volume of tests being performed. Even in a single-physician practice, although you may have an office, will your office manager require (or want) an individual office? Or will a shared office or a designated computer and filing cabinet be sufficient? All things to take into consideration.

AMERICANS WITH DISABILITIES ACT

The Americans with Disabilities Act was enacted in 1990 and has been amended several times, including in January 2009. The Act prohibits discrimination based on disability under specific circumstances. Part of the ADA requires that places of business—including doctors' offices—make reasonable attempts to make their facilities accessible. Exemptions are sometimes made based on remodeling costs and further modified by local building and zoning codes. A rule of thumb is that you are expected to spend 20% of your improvement budget on improved access.

Anyone interested can visit the Americans with Disabilities Act Web site (*www.ada.gov*) and even download a lengthy PDF file on ADA Standards for Accessible Design, which has text, graphics and links to ADA requirements. (*http://www.ada.gov/stdspdf.htm*). Typical requirements are:

- Doors are required to be 26 inches wide and provide a 32-inch opening
- Receptionist counters must accommodate patients in wheelchairs
- Rest rooms need to be wheelchair accessible for both patients and staff
- One exam room should be wheelchair accessible, including the cabinet and under the sink

Again, contractors, designers and architects with experience in designing medical facilities can provide useful ideas. Also, visiting colleagues' offices and asking their staff and your fellow physicians what they like and don't like about their practice spaces can provide real insight into what you need for an efficient, effective space of your own.

> **Action Step:** After hours, with no one in the office, sit in your reception area and view it from different angles to see where changes need to be made. Ask 3 friends in the medical field and 3 outside the medical field to walk through your entire office with a notepad and write down any changes they think could be made to improve aesthetics and better use the space.

ESSENTIAL #27:

Dealing With Stress

How to make sure your job doesn't kill you.

It can be disconcerting to realize that physicians have a higher suicide rate than the general population or other academics. Although that's largely been an anecdotal statement, a paper published in 2004 in the *American Journal of Psychiatry* (Schernhammere ES, Graham AC. Suicide rates among physicians: a quantitative and gender assessment (meta-analysis. *Am J Psychiatry*. 2004;161:2295-2302.) found that male physicians did indeed have a slightly elevated suicide rate and female physicians had a highly elevated suicide rate.

Louise B. Andrew, MD, JD, writing on *eMedicine* in March 2010, cites that "the United States loses the equivalent of at least 1 entire medical school class each year to suicide (reliable estimates are as many as 400 physicians)."

Practicing medicine is a high-stress profession. Although physicians often appear to be in control, that in itself can create stress. And of course, there's a great deal of stress involved in dealing with sick and often dying people on a regular basis. Throw in the complexities and pressures of declining reimbursements, running a business and the potential for devastating lawsuits hanging over your head, and it's not surprising that many physicians have problems with stress that can lead to depression and other health problems, like headaches, upset stomach, rashes, insomnia, ulcers, high blood pressure, heart disease and stroke.

It's hard to define stress, though. What one person finds stressful, another person finds exhilarating. Researchers, however, have tied 85%–90% of all visits to primary care physicians with stress-related conditions. Or put it this way: 112 million people take medication to deal with stress-related symptoms. Here are 10 ways to deal with stress.

1. **Cut the Caffeine.** Yes, start right out with a tough one. But caffeine has been indicted in numerous stress-related conditions. And caffeine is found in coffee, tea, chocolate and colas. These days, even bottled waters and energy drinks are suffused with caffeine. Wean yourself off caffeine gradually, so you don't get withdrawal headaches, then take about 3 weeks to see whether your stress level has decreased. If it has, good; if it hasn't, go back to drinking caffeine if you must and look at other ways to cut stress.

2. **Exercise.** Our reaction to stress, the "fight-or-flight" mechanism, causes our body to react in a way that would precede activity; but mostly we're not in an active mode, we're dealing with patients, staff, endless paperwork or deadlines. Exercising is a logical way to bleed off the excess energy created by stress. Typically, aerobic exercise is recommended for a minimum of 3 times per week for a minimum of 30 minutes each. Aerobic activities include walking, jogging, bicycling, skiing, aerobics, dancing or swimming, among others.

3. **Relaxation and Meditation.** There are a number of different relaxation exercises. For some, it might be medication, self-hypnosis, sitting by a fire, reading a book, lying in a hammock, petting a family pet, sitting by a lake or praying. Some people find reading books or listening to music relaxing.

4. **Sleep.** Nothing can be quite as relaxing as a nap, as long as it's short enough not to screw up your sleep cycle—that usually means 30 minutes or less. If you already struggle with insomnia, it's best to stay away from naps. In addition, most people don't get enough sleep. The average is between 7 and 8 hours of sleep a night. If stress is getting to you, going to bed 30–60 minutes earlier might do the trick.

5. **Leisure and Time-Outs.** Certainly, you've heard that all work and no play made Dr. Jack a dull boy, right? There's a balance that needs to be made—even or especially for physicians—between your work and your play. Everybody needs a break from time to time. The so-called conveniences of the modern age—the Internet, laptop computers, email and smartphones—have made it so easy for us to take our work with us everywhere we go, at home, in the car, on vacation, that we never take time off.

    This can apply to taking a couple 20-minute breaks each day during your workday, or getting out of the office for a walk, run or a visit to the gym; or a longer time, such as a vacation where you don't bring a laptop with you and don't check your email every 15 minutes (or even until you get back home). Generally speaking, the less leisure you have, the higher your stress level.

    Divide your life into 4 segments: Work, family, community and self. (Exclude sleep time.) Now, calculate what percentage of your time you spend on each. There's no normal range, but if you're spending more than 60% of your time on work and less than 10% on self, you might be headed for trouble. Give yourself permission to take a break. Did you know that the word "leisure" is derived from the Old French word "leisir," which means "to be permitted"? Permit yourself some leisure time.

6. **Get Realistic.** Unrealistic expectations cause stress. Expect to make a million dollars your first year in practice? Expect to cure all your patients? Are there areas in your life, whether work or personal, where your expectations are so high that nobody could reach them? Consider adjusting your expectations. Life will be much less stressful.

> *"It's helpful to look at the causes of your stress and decide whether they are really stressful or if it's your reaction to them that's stressful. Some people find roller coasters a thrill; others find them stressful."*

7. **Reframe.** Simply put, reframing can be summed up by the classic question: Is the glass half empty or half full? It's all about perspective and point of view. This can be tough, but it's helpful to look at the causes of your stress and decide whether they are really stressful or if it's your reaction to them that's stressful. Some people find roller

coasters a thrill; others find them stressful. Reframing doesn't change the cause of the stress, but it changes how you perceive it and deal with it.

8. **Beliefs.** This doesn't quite mean your religious or spiritual life, although it can. What this refers to is the many things you believe about life and the way the world and the universe works. If you believe that politicians are all liars, that's a belief that can color all your experiences with government. If you believe that a good father is one who provides for his family, then that colors your experiences and approach to life—and how you perceive yourself. Mostly, we aren't aware of our beliefs because they're so integrated into our ways of thinking.

These belief systems can cause stress, first by the behavior they inspire and, second, by how they conflict with the belief systems of other people. It's amazing how seemingly simple some of these belief systems can be. For instance, perhaps a person believes that in order for a house to be clean, it needs to be vacuumed and dusted every day. That takes up a fair amount of time and a person who thinks once a week is fine doesn't understand why the person who does might feel like a failure (or that the house is a mess) if it isn't thoroughly cleaned daily.

Being aware of our own beliefs and assumptions and restructuring them can go a long way toward decreasing unintentional stress in our lives.

9. **Support System.** Do you deal with stress alone? Or do you share it with someone? Do you have a friend, colleague, religious leader, counselor, spouse or family member you can go to when you're stressed? Sometimes all we need is a listening ear.

10. **Humor.** Laughing relieves tension. Seeing some of the tensions in the world in a humorous light can make dealing with them significantly easier. Laughter, you know, lightens the load. Did you hear the one about the patient who came into the doctor's office with a carrot up his nose, a cucumber in his left ear and a rutabaga in his right ear?

Above all, if the stress is getting to be too much, get help. Don't go it alone. Talk to your own doctor, see a counselor, psychiatrist, psychologist, religious leader or friend. You don't want to be a statistic.

> **Action Step:** One day a month for 12 months, list something you will do to reduce your stress. Each week between that day, write a progress report on how your stress reduction assignment is working.

ESSENTIAL #28:
Effective Patient Scheduling

Tips on managing your caseload.

Who in the White House has more power than the President? The Chief of Staff. Why? Because the Chief of Staff controls the President's schedule—decides who sees him and for how long, who can talk to him on the phone and controls the agenda.

"In the physician's office, the schedule itself is the most powerful
and influential aspect of the physician's day—
and it can control you or you can control it."

In the physician's office, the schedule itself is the most powerful and influential aspect of the physician's day—and it can control you or you can control it. Here are a few thoughts on keeping control of your schedule and making it work for you.

TIME BLOCKS

There is a tendency to let patients decide when they can come into the office. The staff offers a number of open slots, the patient picks one, and that's when they come in. This can lead to a very fragmented schedule.

When possible, try to schedule certain types of procedures in blocks—physicals or new patient appointments on certain days, easy check-ups or procedures opposite more time-consuming procedures, so you can move from 1 room to the next without having a 15-minute lag period after you've seen 1 patient for a 5-minute procedure. This requires that your staff try to determine why the patient is coming in and then slot similar patients in similar ways.

SORTING OUT SAME-DAY PATIENTS

Many offices have problems accommodating "same-day patients," or those patients that call up on the spur of the moment with an emergency. Sometimes these are new patients and they try to accommodate them. This becomes a problem if your schedule is already full and an emergency arises.

One way to deal with this is to leave 1 of the first time slots in the morning open and one of the last morning timeslots open. Do the same thing in the afternoon—an early slot open and a late slot open. Therefore, you have 4 open slots. With the early morning slot, if someone calls first thing in the morning, you can schedule them in, or from the night before, if you have a very late-in-the-day call. If a patient calls later in the morning, you can fit them into the late-morning slot just before lunch, or the just-after-lunch appointment timeslot. Many patients with problems will call during the lunch period, and you can fit them in.

The late-afternoon slot is typically not difficult to fill, because if no emergency is showing up, you can offer it to anyone who calls during the day who is willing to come in on short notice.

It's a good idea, however, to have a written policy in place that discourages habitual same-day callers. Every physician has regular patients whose every concern is an "emergency," even if it's for a routine appointment.

WORK SMARTER

There are several things you can do to help stay on track and work more efficiently. Some of them are really just common sense.

- *Start On Time.* If your first patient is scheduled for 8:00, don't show up at the office at 8:00. Try to get there at least 15 minute early so you can take a breath before plunging into your day. If you run late on your first patient, you'll be behind all day.

- *Chart As You Go.* It's far more efficient to chart as you go along, either dictating between rooms, while in the room or by having a charting system in the rooms so you can chart during the examination. There are a lot of good reasons for this, but one of the most important is that you'll make fewer mistakes and forget fewer details if you don't wait for later in the day—or week—to write up your notes on a patient.

- *Schedule Breaks.* It's easy to get into a habit of taking breaks between patients, even if it's for a few minutes—chat for a minute with a staffer, have a cup of coffee, check your email or your Facebook page, make a personal phone call. But think about it this way: If you take a 3-minute break between each patient and you see 5 patients an hour over 8 hours, you've just wasted 2 hours of your day. Better to schedule a break to get these minor tasks done and control the time than watch it add up like a drippy sink.

> *"Think about it this way: If you take a 3-minute break between each patient and you see 5 patients an hour over 8 hours, you've just wasted 2 hours of your day."*

- *Set Targets.* To get a real handle on your scheduling, you need to set a target number of patients per day based on the number of hours available. This helps in setting expected revenue goals. Once you have that number, you need to evaluate your no-shows and late cancellations. Whoever on your staff is assigned the responsibility of scheduling also needs to know what those per-day patient goals are and commit to meeting them.

- *Keep Busy.* Evaluate your daily routine. Are there periods when you have nothing to do or when there are no patients scheduled? Why? Is it intentional? Necessary? If not, can you organize your schedule to accommodate work-related activities? Having a sense of what's going on in your day on a regular basis will go a long way toward how to approach your patient scheduling.

> **Action Step:** Ask each of your front office and clinical team members to make a list of 5 ways they feel you can more effectively schedule your patients. For 1 month, perform a Time and Motion study, analyzing the flow of your staff and patients, then develop a plan to improve the patient flow.

Tips For Collecting Money Owed

Dealing with delinquent accounts.

Very few physicians that go into private practice realize they have just added a very unpleasant line to their resume—collection agency. It's certainly not something taught in medical school. But the fact is, anyone who is self-employed, whether running a physician's office or a construction company, will, from time to time, have to go after the money; and, unfortunately, will occasionally not get paid for their services.

Patients that don't pay typically fall into 3 categories:

1. Patients who don't pay
2. Patients who can't pay
3. Patients who won't pay

Each of these types presents unique problems. Not all of these problems will have solutions. **Patients that don't pay** generally do not have an explanation, but there may be several reasons for their delinquency. Only a small portion of patients who don't pay can't pay or won't pay. Determining the cause of their lack of payment allows you to solve it.

Patients who can't pay, typically because of financial issues, present a unique set of issues for physicians. Most businesses will just not extend services to customers who can't afford to pay for those services. In medicine, this can present a moral dilemma. Can you continue to provide care?

Patients who won't pay can afford to pay, but have chosen not to. There may be a variety of reasons for this, which we will address, but these are almost always the most difficult delinquent patients to deal with.

> *"Part of the image we want to project is that of diligent medical professionals; how you handle your financial affairs needs to send and project that same message."*

PATIENTS WHO DON'T PAY

Patients who don't pay are sending you a message. Determining what that message is leads to potential solutions. One simple reason is: Perhaps they never received the bill. Maybe they've forgotten it or lost it. This means you and your staff will have to go after the money, and the key to that is communication. Part of the image we want to project is that of diligent medical professionals; how you handle your financial affairs needs to send and project that same message.

A trained member of your staff should initiate contact with the patient. This person needs people skills and a complete list of responses to the most common excuses non-paying patients will offer. The staffer needs to remain calm and professional—no anger, cynicism or sarcasm.

Sometimes it's more effective—not easier, but more effective—to schedule a meeting with the patient to come into the office and discuss their nonpayment in person.

Phone calls should be approached as follows:

- Start by reminding the patient that they have an unpaid bill. (Have a copy available.)
- Confirm that the patient received the bill. If not, confirm their address.
- Politely ask when your office can expect the payment. Offer to collect the balance using a credit card. Offer a payment fee if applicable.
- Listen attentively, not just to the words, but to the patient's inflection and emotional response.
- Be polite, yet firm and professional.
- Try to determine if the patient actually intends to pay the bill.
- If the patient does not intend to pay the bill, try to decide whether this is a **can't pay** or a **won't pay** situation.
- Keep track of patients who say they will pay. If they can't or won't, you want to know that as soon as possible.

If your own practice has a large proportion of patients who don't pay their bills, you need to evaluate your billing process. Flexibility in payment is important: Accept credit cards and payment plans. Many practices include a "rebilling charge" that adds $10 or $15 each month to a patient's bill when the first invoice is ignored. This is simpler than charging interest, which requires additional tax forms and accountings.

PATIENTS WHO CAN'T PAY

Patients who can't pay, typically because of financial hardship, present a real difficulty. Most physicians are willing to perform a certain amount of pro bono medical work. Pro bono work is typically recognized as an important part of a physician's professional obligation. Nonetheless, you have to be careful just how much nonpaying work you do, or you will go out of business or find yourself offering substandard care. Also, generally speaking, you'll find it a much more rewarding experience to choose the pro bono care you offer, rather than having it thrust upon you.

If a patient has a history of on-time payments and they're temporarily having financial difficulties, that may be enough cause for taking on their care while their problems are sorted out.

For new patients, one of the keys is to establish a patient's payment history or financial resources. Consider performing a credit check on new patients. This is a common practice in most other areas of business. Information necessary for a financial check is current employer and income, bank accounts and balances, credit card and loan balances, outstanding taxes and so on. If you're going to provide pro bono work or offer extended credit to a patient, it's well worth your time and resources to decide why and what your own risk is. You then have to balance that information with a moral judgment about the care the patient requires.

PATIENTS WHO WON'T PAY

These are by far the most difficult patients to deal with. Some are simply scam artists and your medical practice is probably not the first business they have stiffed on payment. There's only one way to deal with these people: Say, "No, thank you."

The rest of the "won't pay" patients are typically making some sort of statement about your bill and their feelings about the value of your services, your skills or your relationship with them. It's usually not about the cost of your services, but value, or perceived value. This comes down to trust and respect.

If patients trust and respect you and the medical care you provide, they are more likely to value the relationship, which results in on-time payments. When you decide that a patient is a "won't pay" patient, it's important to communicate with them to determine what it is about your services or you that they are unhappy with. Generally, this discussion should be face-to-face. It's important to remember that this is less about getting the bill paid than it is about reestablishing a trusting relationship with a patient.

- Ask the patient to help you understand the problem with the relationship and the service.
- Let the patient know you value them and the relationship.
- Let the patient know you want to try and salvage the real or perceived problem.
- Listen.
- If the patient does not want to talk, try to draw them out with nondefensive questions like "What went wrong?" or "What aspects of your care do you think could be improved?"

Once you find out what the problem is, you need to determine if it's possible to fix it. Is it a real problem? Do the patient's claims have merit? Will it be possible to save the relationship? Continue care or inform the patient they will need to find a different physician? If you do continue, can you get assurances that you'll receive payment?

Once you've determined that improvements can be made and what they are, discuss how you will deal with the outstanding fees. Ask them how they would like to pay the outstanding invoice. If this doesn't work to either party's satisfaction, discuss terminating the relationship. Keep it professional and calm. Offer to help them find a new physician, if necessary.

Then follow up on the fee again. Unless the problem is clearly your fault, do not agree to a direct reduction in your fee—patients view this as a sign of guilt or weakness. Send the patient a certified letter with the reasons for ending the relationship spelled out and provide a grace period for urgent or emergency care (45–90 days is typical).

EXAMPLE OF A PATIENT COLLECTION TIMETABLE

Day 1

- Submit the CMS-1500 claim to the appropriate payer by mail or electronically. Collect balances, co-pay and coinsurance at the time of service.

Day 30

- Review each account. If payment has not been received, telephone the carrier. Make certain you get the name of the person you are speaking with and ask for the claim status. Ask when payment should be expected.
- If the carrier has not received the claim, confirm the address and refile the claim; make it to the attention of the person you spoke with earlier. Ask if you may fax it as soon as possible for their immediate attention.
- Verify the new claim has been received.
- Send out patient invoices for all patient balances.

Day 60

- Send out a letter to the patient stating that payment has not been received from the carrier and that your practice is requesting assistance in obtaining payment.
- If the patient still owes a balance, call the patient to confirm their address and verify they received the invoices. Ask why the previous invoice was not paid. Ask when payment can be expected.
- Request credit card payment.

Day 75

- Phone the patient to discuss required payment arrangements. Send the patient a written confirmation of any agreement made.

Day 90

- Send the patient a past-due letter indicating the consequences for nonpayment according to the signed financial policy. Send a copy of the signed financial policy.

Day 120

- Send a final collection letter to the patient via certified mail. Follow up with a telephone call.
- Prepare the account for outside collection or civil action if no payment is received within 72 hours.

Action Steps:

1. Create a step-by-step protocol for how your office will deal with collecting money owed by patients from the minute they make an appointment to the minute they make payment at the front desk.

2. Develop short and simple scripts for your staff to say when:
   — they are telling patients that a balance is due when presenting to the office front desk
   — the patient says that they do not have their co-pay today
   — the patient says "I am out of work and have a difficult time paying the bill"
   — patients indicate they were not happy with the service they are being asking to pay fors

Dealing With The Difficult Patient

More tips on effective communication and dealing with the toughest patients.

Every physician deals with a range of personalities. Every physician can cite difficult patients; most often, difficult patients fall under the "noncompliant" label. It is possible to turn a bad patient into a good patient, and what it requires is effective communication.

All patients want to feel important—to be acknowledged, feel appreciated and be valued.

We can start by how we enter the patient room. Remember your body language. You have about 60 seconds to make a lasting impression. According to UCLA researcher Dr. Albert Mahrabian, 55% of effective communication is nonverbal; 38% is tone of voice; 7% is verbal. So remember to:

- Make eye contact
- Have a friendly demeanor
- Smile
- Make a connecting comment.

Not only does this break the ice, but it puts you in control of the encounter.

According to social and psychological studies, people make an average of 11 decisions about you in the first 7 seconds of contact. Within 4 minutes, they've made a decision on whether to continue or break off the relationship.

To get off to a good start, in addition to body language, your first communication after a greeting is to indicate that you have the patient's best interests at heart and intend to provide complete and high-quality care. Say something along the lines of, "Today, we want to make sure we find out what you have, why you have it, your options for treatment, and that you understand the treatment plan."

> *"To get off to a good start, in addition to body language, your first communication after a greeting is to indicate that you have the patient's best interests at heart and intend to provide complete and high-quality care."*

Part of this strategy is to co-opt the patient's cooperation and make them a partner in their care and treatment.

Before you leave, shake hands, make eye contact and thank them for coming in. Tell them to call you if they have more questions or concerns.

NONCOMPLIANCE

There are at least 7 reasons for a patient's noncompliance:

1. They do not believe they need care
2. Language barriers
3. They believe the care is too expensive
4. They don't understand the treatment plan
5. Undesirable side effects
6. Personal conflicts with the provider
7. Philosophical, cultural or religious beliefs.

When dealing with a noncompliant patient, it is important to respond, not react. Responding involves understanding the reasons behind a patient's noncompliance and acting accordingly. Reacting does not involve thought or planning, and often becomes negative and adversarial.

> *"When dealing with a noncompliant patient, it is important to respond, not react. Responding involves understanding the reasons behind a patient's noncompliance and acting accordingly. Reacting does not involve thought or planning and often becomes negative and adversarial."*

To respond, you need to listen to what a patient is actually saying and determine why they are saying it.

It's important to project warmth, friendliness and understanding. It's even better to *feel* warmth, friendliness and understanding. Yes, that can be tough for some patients, but understanding and empathy can go a long way toward developing those attitudes toward even the most difficult patients.

Here are 5 steps for accomplishing that objective.

1. *Show Respect.* Although this seems obvious, it can sometimes be difficult, particularly if a patient is being rude or disagreeable. Ultimately, the key is to maintain the dignity of the patient. The patient has the right to choose or refuse treatment.
2. *Practice Active Listening.* Ask open-ended questions in order to draw out the person. Respond to the patient regularly so they know you're listening. Use lead-in phrases like, "Help me understand why you aren't following through with our treatment plan." We need to not just gather information, but try to understand the emotions of the patients.
3. *Show Concern.* Learn to express concern appropriately. Patients perceive caring by how we respond to them, when we make eye contact, our body language and tone of voice. Lean forward slightly to show you're paying attention; avoid crossing your arms, which is perceived as closed-off and close-minded; nod your head and use facial expressions that demonstrate your concern. Use tactful and appropriate touch, placing a hand on

the patient's arm or foot for a brief moment. Monitor the patient's reaction to the touch and withdraw if the patient responds negatively.

4. *Be Objective.* Like responding vs reacting, in dealing with a noncompliant or difficult patient, it's important that we keep our emotions under control. Don't jump to conclusions; gather as many facts as possible. If you get angry and speak sharply, there's every likelihood that the patient will respond in a similar fashion, mirroring your behavior.

5. *Accept the Patient.* Let's face it; no one's going to like every patient. But it's possible to accept the patient while not accepting their behavior. Learn to recognize when your problem is with the patient's personality rather than their behavior and to understand what behavior you're not going to be able to change.

Sometimes patients are just plain difficult. They have negative personalities and they approach life in a combative way. Here are some tips for dealing with these patients:

- Remember that sometimes it's pointless to argue. The patient may be insecure. Go with the flow.
- Don't push. It will only escalate the conflict.
- Notice if their problems are made worse by stress. A tactical retreat may be in order so you can regroup and try again at a better time.
- Don't beat up on yourself. Respond instead of react and don't blame yourself.

Sometimes it's appropriate to apologize. There can be some issues with saying you're sorry. Malpractice insurers often insist that an apology is an admission of guilt, fault or negligence that will increase the risk of litigation. Some insurers will even void a malpractice policy if the physician apologizes to a patient after a complication or error.

However, there have been a number of studies that point out that there is an inverse relationship between being sued and communication skills: the odds of being sued go down as communication skills increase. Another study suggests that the likelihood of a lawsuit decreases by 50% if an apology is made along with timely release of the details of the medical error.

Dr. Michael Woods, author of *Healing Words—The Power of Apology in Medicine*, points out 5 reasons to apologize:

1. Shows patients respect
2. Shows you're taking responsibility for the problem
3. Shows you care about the patient's feelings
4. Shows your empathy
5. Diffuses anger and disarms the patient

It also is likely to diffuse tension and stress caused by the medical error.

In his book, Woods goes on to discuss what he calls the 4 R's of an apology. They are:

- *Recognition.* You need to recognize your own emotions as well as the feelings of the patient and family. If you feel genuinely guilty about an error, there's a good likelihood that an apology is appropriate.

- *Regret.* Expressing regret shows you have empathy for the patient's situation and that you feel bad about it. Say something along the lines of "I'm very sorry. I understand this outcome was not what you or I expected." This doesn't express guilt, but can lead toward healing.
- *Responsibility.* By apologizing, you're taking ownership and responsibility of the problem.
- *Remedy.* It's important to supply a solution to the problem caused by the error.

Effective communication is the key. Being a caregiver requires being an effective communicator.

> **Action Step:** Think of a real situation that you experienced with a difficult patient and outline what you would now do differently. Ask all on your team to do the same, and have an office meeting to review as a group and discuss better ways to deal with difficult patients.

Balancing Your Personal And Professional Lives

Business might be good, but there's more to life.

Money isn't everything. You could work a hundred hours a week and earn a ton of money, but would you want to?

Part of the key is to be efficient. Analyzing how you're spending your time often reveals that you're just plain wasting time on non–money-making tasks—talking on the phone with your broker, taking personal phone calls, checking your Facebook page, chatting too much with staff or patients. That isn't to say you can't do some of that, but some physicians find that once they get control of those things they have as much as 20% more time in the day to either see patients or enjoy life.

Unfortunately, although practicing medicine can be a gratifying, rewarding profession, for many physicians it's an increasingly stressful job filled with increasingly unpleasant busywork that doesn't add anything to the bottom line.

Sometimes the answer is: Work a little less.

> *"Although practicing medicine can be a gratifying, rewarding*
> *profession, for many physicians it's an increasingly stressful job*
> *filled with increasingly unpleasant busywork*
> *that doesn't add anything to the bottom line.*
> *"Sometimes the answer is: Work a little less."*

Work a little less and walk into the office a happier human being. If you're a happier human being, you'll produce more money and your staff will be happier.

What follows are 23 steps to balancing your personal and professional life.

1. *Lifelong Learning.* Remain a student. Make a commitment to education, formal or informal. A medical career is not a destination, it's a journey. Take the time to learn new things.

2. *Be Ethical.* In a 2008 report in the *Archives of Pediatric Adolescent Medicine*, it was reported that 44.7% of survey participants felt that their ethics education during medical residency was fair or poor. That's rather sad, isn't it? Because the medical profession involves facing ethical questions every single day. Typically, the best ethical response is to do what is in the best interest of the patient. Many state medical licensing boards require continual medical education courses in ethics. Think of it as an opportunity, not a burden.

3. *Don't Be Too Efficient.* Physicians are not robots. Sometimes the best thing you can do is listen to a patient, even if it takes a couple minutes out of your schedule. This interaction can be a surprisingly enriching experience—for you!

4. *Leave It At Work.* At the end of your workday, write down the things that really bugged you. Then leave the list—and your issues—at the office and go home.

5. *Take Control Of Your Finances.* How much debt do physicians leave medical school with? $250,000? $500,000? A lot. So, clearly, when you start out, you have a lot of debt to pay off. But learn to save as well. You want financial security at the end of your career, when you can truly enjoy practicing medicine, not because you're paying bills.

6. *Learn To Say "No."* The road to burnout is paved with saying "Yes" to everything. It is possible to take on too many projects or accept too many responsibilities. Before you accept, ask yourself: Will it enhance my career? Will it take away from my time with family and friends? Will it lead to balance or imbalance in my life? Sometimes the best possible answer is "No."

7. *Prioritize.* Have you ever thought about the epitaph that will be written on your tombstone? Have you ever seen one that said, "He sure spent a lot of time at the office"? No. It's about being a good parent or a loved one. People on their deathbeds don't wish they'd spent more time at work. They wished they'd spent more time with family and friends. In order to have balance in your life, you need to remember that.

8. *Accept Your Limitations.* Doctors can't save all patients. Doctors can't do everything. Sometimes your to-do list just won't be completed. Accept it and move on.

9. *Vacation.* Take days off on a regular basis. Do it often enough and regularly enough that your staff and patients become used to the idea. Let yourself become accustomed to the idea without guilt.

10. *Find A Niche.* What do you most want to do as a physician? What are you best at? Focus on that. Focusing your energies on a single area of expertise or interest can lead to amazing success.

11. *Spread Out Your Interactions.* Sometimes it seems like we get into the habit of spending time with people our same age starting in kindergarten. But once we're out of school, there's a great deal of enrichment that can come from spending time with people younger and older than yourself.

12. *Exceed Patients' Expectations.* There's great pleasure to be found in going the extra mile for patients. Your patients will remember you for it and keep coming back.

13. *Ask: What Do You Need?* Ask your family and staff what they need most from you. Their answers might surprise you.

14. *No Work Talk!* When you're socializing with other physicians, try to talk about something other than medicine. Yes, there's a whole wide world out there.

15. *Don't Procrastinate.* Clean up your inbox, prioritize your tasks, break them down into manageable chunks, complete medical records before they pile up. Respond to emails

quickly and efficiently, return phone calls in a timely fashion. Be a disciplined doctor and a decider, not a procrastinator.

16. *Multitask.* Except when you need to really concentrate on one thing with all your focus and attention. And learn to tell which is which.

17. *Dine Together.* Eat at least 1 meal a day with family or friends.

18. *Create A Support System.* Nobody performs well in a vacuum. Everybody needs somebody who will listen to us, who understands us better than we understand ourselves, somebody who can say, "You really need a vacation," or "You're under too much stress; take a break."

19. *Take Weekends Off—When You Can.* When you're not scheduled to work, take the weekend off . . . and don't work. Don't go into the office to get caught up—you rarely do. Tell friends and family what you're trying to do so they can help you break the habit.

20. *Make Non-doctor Friends.* Yes, make friends with people who are not physicians, nurses and who don't want you to be their doctor.

21. *Be Flexible.* Balance is a shifting concept. Stress and busy periods are a part of any career, but learning to balance it and deal with it is the key to survival.

22. *Take Your Own Road.* Everybody's journey through life is different. What works for one doesn't necessarily work for another. Recognize that the challenges you face are yours alone and, although they may be shared, they're unique to you. Try to pause and enjoy the journey along the way, because it is unique to you.

23. *Have Fun.* Take your profession seriously, but use some humor. Smile. Laugh. Enjoy what you're doing.

> **Action Step:** Make a list of 5 things you would like to do more often. Review daily and little by little begin to do more of those activities, explaining to family, coworkers and friends your mission. Keep a daily log to list activities that you start to spend more time on from your list.
> Read a book called *One Minute For Yourself* by Spencer Johnson.

Action Plan

#1. Craft your mission statement. Schedule a 2-hour meeting with your office team to assist in developing your office mission statement, so everyone will have ownership in it. Display it on all written practice materials. Frame and hang your mission statement in your reception area, break room and other key areas.

#2. List the benefits of your current location (or future office site) and how those benefits will be used in your strategic plan. If you plan to move to a new location or start in practice, list the pros and cons of locations you are considering.

#3. Create a business plan as discussed in Essential #3, focusing on areas of your practice that need growth or improvement. Be specific, and have action plans and plans for regular monitoring.

#4. Speak to your accountant and discuss which corporate structure would be best for you based on your current needs and plans for future growth, both professionally and personally.

#5. Create an annual practice budget, including all key areas, and review it with your accountant. A good exercise to do while working on your budget is to look for areas for cost containment with a solid plan to reduce costs in those areas. Creativity is the key.

#6. Determine your optimum staffing in each area of your office—front office, clinical, back office and billing. Create an interview protocol and questions to use for future recruiting. Be as detailed as possible. Make a list of mistakes you have made in the past when interviewing.

#7. List personality traits you possess that will make you a good leader and write your plans for the next 12 months, which should be reviewed on a regular basis. Ask everyone in your office to anonymously write what they feel your strengths and weaknesses are as a leader (and be sure to have tissues in hand!).

#8. Along with key team members, create your marketing budget and plan, focusing on both patient retention and development. What are your chief weaknesses in internal and external marketing? List 3 ways to improve them.

#9. Craft (or update) your office manual. Ask 1 or 2 physicians in your area if you can review their office manuals for ideas on how to improve yours.

#10. List 5–10 changes that you and your team can make immediately to enhance your efficiency. Be sure to take baby steps or little may change.

#11. Plan 1 motivational action for (each employee this month) each of the next 3 months. List the 10 simple things you can do to motivate and thank your office team.

#12. Take steps this month (trade shows, online, etc) to perform due diligence on EHR implementation. Create a simple written plan on how you are planning to begin EHR usage. Set goals relating to this with a timeline and stick to it!

#13. List ways in which technology might enhance your out-of-the-office productivity. What new systems do you want to implement to increase efficiency and save time when away from the office? Can any of this technology help anyone else on your office team?

#14. Investigate, set up and utilize e-prescribing within the next 6 months. Write a timeline and steps necessary for the implementation and decide who on your office team will be responsible for each step.

#15. Measure and monitor billing/collections strengths and weaknesses quarterly and compare to industry benchmarks. List pros and cons of switching the way you do billing (in-house vs a billing service) and if there is a significant reason for changing. If so, list action items for possible change.

#16. Monitor your practice data monthly, quarterly and annually. Create simple spread-sheets for assessment and identify areas of concern. Write action plans for improvement. Appoint appropriate team members to help with each of these areas.

#17. List 5 strategies that will reduce your expenses over the next 12 months. Blend these strategies together with the Action Step from Essential #3, and make sure they become part of your budget projections.

#18. List 1 new service that your practice will provide within the next 12 months and cite your plan for implementation. Do this exercise on an annual basis.

#19. List 3 products that you can immediately begin to dispense in your office. List how you plan to train your office team in presenting these products to your patients and develop treatment protocols for their use. Integrate 2–3 new products every 6 months with the same plan.

#20. Create effective scripts for your 5 most frequent patient dialogues, for both the front office and the clinical team. Practice the scripts regularly at special office meetings. Add 5 new scripts monthly until all are completed.

#21. List 2 collection strategies for your front office team and also your billing team that you will employ this year to boost your revenue.

#22. Create an activity log to assess how you spend your time over a 14-day period. List 3 things over a 1-month period that you can do in order to optimize your time. Then, 1 month later, do the same exercise. Keep a daily log of 1 thing you do for yourself that is important to you. It can be simple.

#23. List what factors in your practice and personal life that could initiate consideration of an associate. Knowing your current situation, develop a timeframe for those factors.

#24. Review your medical malpractice policy to be sure you are covered appropriately in all areas and get an estimate from 1 other medical malpractice insurance company.

#25. After hours, with no one in the office, sit in your reception area and view it from different angles to see where changes need to be made. Ask 3 friends in the medical field and 3 outside the medical field to walk through your entire office with a notepad and write down any changes they think could be made to improve aesthetics and better use the space.

#26. One day a month for 12 months, list something you will do to reduce your stress. Each week between that day, write a progress report on how your stress reduction assignment is working.

#27. Ask each of your front office and clinical team members to make a list of 5 ways they feel you can more effectively schedule your patients. For 1 month, perform a Time and Motion study, analyzing the flow of your staff and patients, then develop a plan to improve the patient flow.

#28. Create a step-by-step protocol for how your office will deal with collecting money owed by patients from the minute they make an appointment to the minute they make payment at the front desk. Develop short and simple scripts for your staff to say when:
— they are telling patients that a balance is due when presenting to the office front desk
— the patient says that they do not have their co-pay today
— the patient says "I am out of work and have a difficult time paying the bill"
— patients indicate they were not happy with the service they are being asking to pay for

#29. Think of a real situation that you experienced with a difficult patient and outline what you would now do differently. Ask all on your team to do the same, and have an office meeting to review as a group and discuss better ways to deal with difficult patients.

#30. Make a list of 5 things you would like to do more often. Review daily and little by little begin to do more of those activities, explaining to family, coworkers and friends your mission. Keep a daily log to list activities that you start to spend more time on from your list. Read a book called *One Minute For Yourself* by Spencer Johnson.

Afterword

The Essentials outlined in this book can make you a better physician and help you run your practice in a more efficient way, hopefully resulting in a happier, more financially stable you. Through decades of running our own practices and helping other physicians with theirs, we have boiled down the essentials into this book. But finally, at the end of each day, we suggest you create a personal checklist that you look at. Here's ours:

- [ ] Did I read my personal mission statement today?
- [ ] Did I read my goal list today?
- [ ] Did I compliment 3 people today?
- [ ] Did I tell my staff how much I appreciate them today?
- [ ] Did I send a thank-you note to at least 1 person for helping me and my practice?
- [ ] Did I see all of my patients within 15 minutes of their scheduled times?
- [ ] Did I do 1 thing that brought me closer to my goals and objectives today?
- [ ] Did I do my dictation on every patient today?
- [ ] Did I maintain eye contact and smile when entering each treatment room today?
- [ ] Did I thank every patient for coming to the office today?
- [ ] Did I ask patients about their family and friends, and suggest that they see their doctors for preventive health care?
- [ ] Did I ask each patient about having any additional questions?
- [ ] Did I remain positive and motivated toward everyone I met today?
- [ ] Did I tell my children and spouse that I love them today?
- [ ] Did I read my "Did I?" list every evening and morning?

Well, did you?

APPENDIX:
Benchmarks And Equations

I. Determining Office Size and Proportions

Rule of thumb: 1,200–1,500 square feet for the first physician; add 1,000–1,200 square feet for each additional physician, up to 4 or 5 physicians.

A traditional 1-physician office would have 3 exam rooms, a consultation room, a reception room, and a business office and/or storage space.

If you have more exam rooms, you can have a smaller reception room. To calculate, consider your busiest hour and figure the number of patients you expect to see during that time period. Multiply that number by 2.5. This accounts not just for patients, but parents of children or relatives and friends who may accompany the patient. Subtract the number of exam rooms. This gives you the number of chairs.

For example, 10 patients × 2.5 = 25–3 exam rooms = 22 chairs.

Multiply the number of chairs by 20 square feet.

22 chairs × 20 square feet = 240 square feet for your reception room.

II. Per Patient Visit Calculations

For the sake of simplicity, you've looked up your per patient revenue average through your professional organization and it is $100 per patient per visit. In order for you to meet your $21,000 monthly budget, you will need to have 210 patient visits per month.

From that point, you now know how many patients you need through your door and the average amount of income per patient you need to generate. Now you can create a somewhat circular equation to determine if you have enough money in your practice budget to make contacts and develop referral sources in order to generate 210 patients per month through advertising, marketing and communication.

Other cost factors you will need to consider are repairs and maintenance, postage, contract management services, billing (in-house vs contracting outside), security, disposal of medical waste, telephone, cell phone expenses, Internet expenses, etc.

III. Budget Percentages

There are loose percentage benchmarks that you can expect to hit in your total budget, although it will vary from specialty to specialty. For instance, in podiatry, we generally expect 20%–25% of the budget to go toward salaries, wages and benefits; 5%–7% to go toward rent; 2%–3% to go toward advertising; 8%–10% for medical supplies; and 3%–4% for office supplies.

IV. Number of Staff

If you're starting your practice, hiring a lot of people right from the get-go can also be cost-prohibitive. Many practice management consultants recommend beginning with an office manager and possibly 1 technician and a medical assistant or nurse. If you perform surgery in your practice, you may need more core staff. Typically, most consultants suggest 3½ staff per physician.

Another rule of thumb is you need 1½ front office staff for every 1 back office staff.

Another way of determining number of staff involves looking at money. In this case, typical medical practices function best when their payroll ratio is 20%–22%. That is to say: Payroll and whatever health benefits or other benefits you intend to provide make up 20%–22% of the amount of collections annually. If you expect your practice to bring in $1,000,000 annually, then your payroll should be around $200,000–$220,000.

That is just for support staff and doesn't include your salary.

V. Marketing Budget

Although how much of your budget should go to marketing varies from consultant to consultant, a general rule of thumb is 10% of your projected revenues should be set aside from marketing.

VI. Per Visit Value

We think a significantly more important benchmark is the per visit value (PVV). The PVV is determined by dividing total collections by total patient visits:

(Total Collections/Total Patient Visits = Per Visit Value)

The average PVV will vary depending on specialty. For instance, in podiatry, the number you see cited the most is $99, although some sources cite $90.

Although this is a very basic benchmark, it's one that has ramifications in every type of business, whether it's an online business (Per Click Value) or a restaurant (Per Customer Value), etc. PVV provides a value of how productive you are.

However, because we're physicians, it doesn't always come down to a dollar amount. You need to look at what you're doing for each patient—not just injections, not just visits or ancillary care, but vascular testing, neurological testing, physical therapy in your office and dispensing products in-office.

VII. Payroll Ratio

Payroll ratio is calculated by taking your total staff payroll—not just salary of support staff, but the salaries and payroll taxes and benefits, like 401Ks, and totaling them (for just the support staff)—and dividing that number by annual collections. This provides the payroll ratio and, if your practice is operating efficiently, it should be somewhere between 22%–26% of collections.

(Total Staff Payroll/Annual Collections = Payroll Ratio)

VIII. Accounts Receivable

Accounts receivable (A/R) will also vary from practice specialty to practice specialty, but one rule of thumb is that a practice's total accounts receivable is <2 months worth of gross charges. For example, if your practice is billing $65,000 per month, the practice should have a total A/R of less than $130,000. In addition, you will want <15% of the total accounts receivable to be 90 days outstanding.

IX. Days in Receivables

This particular benchmark can be taken one step further, to *days in receivables*, which is defined as how long the average claim takes to be paid. The equation for that is:

$$([\text{Total Accounts Receivable}/\text{Gross Annual Charges}] \times 365 = \text{Days in Receivables})$$

X. Associate Salary Calculations

The most common method is a *base salary plus an incentive*, which shares the risk between the senior partner (you) and the associate. The associate is paid a nominal base salary and receives a bonus after a specific preset level of income is generated. Our recommendation is that the income threshold be approximately 3 times the associate's base salary. For example, if you decide the base salary is $50,000 annually, the associate is rewarded a bonus starting when they have generated $150,000 of practice income.

Typically, a percentage of each dollar made above that threshold payment is awarded, usually 15%–25%. So, once the associate brings in $150,000 of revenue to the practice, they start earning 15–25 cents on every dollar they bring in. This bonus can be calculated and paid out monthly or quarterly. The advantages of this system are that it gives the associate continual feedback as well as incentives and active participation in the practice's financial health.

A

Access control, security, 54–55

Accounts receivable
    assessment, 67
    benchmark, 135

Action plan, 127–129

Active listening, 81, 120

ADA Standards for Accessible Design, 103

Advertising costs, 70

Advice sheets, 90

Aerobic exercise, 105

Affiliations, 25

Age, prospective employee's, 25

American Academy of Family Physicians (AAFP), 43

American Journal of Psychiatry, 105

Americans with Disabilities Act, 103

Ancillary services, 73–76

Andrew, Louise B., 105

Antikickback statute, Medicare, 75–76

Appointments

online scheduling, 51
    schedule planning, 45
    staying on track, 89

Arrest record, 25

Ash, Mary Kay, 83

Assessments, practice, 65–68

Associates
    adding, 93–96
    salary calculations, 135

Association, 82

Association of Health Care Office Management, 29

Authentication, 55

Automobile insurance, 98

B

Back office staff, 22

Balancing personal and professional lives, 123–125

Beliefs, 107

Benchmarks, 67–68, 133–135

Billing
    accounts receivable, 67, 135
    benchmarks, 135
    collecting money, 86
    company versus in-house billing, 61–64
    online, 52

Body language, 119, 120–121
Breaktime, 110
Brochures, 37
Budgeting, 10–11, 17–20
   cutting, 69
   marketing, 134
   percentages benchmark, 133
Business description
   marketing plan, 35
   writing, 9–10
Business income interruption insurance, 97–98
Business plan, 9–14
Buying equipment, 70

C
Caffeine, 105
Caretools, 53–54
C corp, 16
Certification Commission for Healthcare Information Technology (CCHIT), 52
Chairs, reception area size and, 8
Charting, maintaining, 110
Checklists, 46
Citizenship, 25
Client satisfaction assessment, 66
Clinical Laboratory Improvement Amendments (CLIA), 74
Collecting revenue, 86
Collection work, 113–117
Communication
   collecting payment, 113–115
   difficult patients, 119–122
   office dynamics, 45
   with patients, 81–83
Commuting time, 5
Competition, tracking, 32
Compliance, patients', 81–82
Comprehensive general liability insurance, 97
Computer use, 51–52
   auditing systems, 86
   corporation, setting up, 16
   electronic medical records and electronic health records, 52, 59
   e-prescribing, 52, 57–60
   hiring consideration, 23
   remote access, 53–55
Confidentiality protocol, 43
Continuity, referring physicians, 32–33

Contrast, 82

Controlled substances, 60

Corporate structure, 15–16

Costs

    advertising, 70

    electronic health records (EHR), 59

    equipment, 70

    managed care, 65

    overhead, 69–71

    per-patient, calculating, 13–14

    telephone services, 70

CVS Caremark Corporation, 58

D

Days in receivables, 135

Deaths from medication errors, 57

Decisiveness, 81

Delegating responsibility, 91

Department of Health and Human Services (DHHS), 52

Description, business

    marketing plan, 35

    writing, 9–10

Device control, security, 54

Dictation, 90

Difficult patients, 119–122

Disabilities, 25

Disability insurance, 98–99

The Doorknob Moment, 83

Drug Enforcement Agency (DEA) limits on e-prescribing, 60

E

Effectiveness, 45–46

Efficiency, 101–102

    office design, 101–102

    staff, 45–46

Electronic health records (EHR), 52

    cost of, 59

    e-prescribing, 57, 58

Electronic medical records (EMR), 52

Emotions, keeping under control, 121

Employees. *See* Staff

Employment-related practices insurance, 99–100

E-newsletters, 39

Entity authentication, 55

Epocrates, Inc., 53, 54

E-prescribing computer programs, 57–60
Equations
   days in receivables, 135
   payroll ratio, 134
   per visit value (PVV), 134
Equipment
   ancillary service, 46, 74, 103
   budgeting, 17
   costs, 11, 65, 70
Ethics, 123
Exam rooms, 101
Exercise, managing stress, 105
Express Scripts, Inc., 58

F
Family status, 25
FedEx Corporation mission statement, 2–3
Feedback, 92, 96
Finances
   budgeting, 10–11, 17–20
   cutting expenses, 69
   percentages benchmark, 133
Financial hardships, patients with, 114–115
Financial soundness assessment, 65
Front office staff, 22

G
Giannulli, Dr. Thomas, 53–54
Gifts, 31, 32
Goals, financial incentives tied to, 47–48
Government regulations
   antikickback statute, 75–76
   Drug Enforcement Agency (DEA) limits on e-prescribing, 60
   e-prescribing, 57–58, 59
   following up, 87
   HIPAA laws, 43, 54–55
   interviewing prospective employees, 25
Guiliana, John, mission statement, 3

H
Harassment lawsuits, 100
Health benefits, 22
   listing in office manual, 41–42
   pay structure with and without, 19–20
HIPAA laws, 43, 54–55

Hiring staff, 21–25

Hospital, relationship with, 12–13

Humor, 107

I

IChart, 53–54

Illegal job interview questions, 24–25

Incentives

   associate, 135

   employee, 47–48

   e-prescribing, 59

   marketing, 39

In-office dispensing, 77–79

Insurance companies, medical

   following up, 87

   marketing, 13–14

   online confirmation, 52

Insuring your business, 97–100

Internal marketing, 37–38

Internet. *See also* Web site

   appointment scheduling, 51

   assessing use of, 40

   billing and insurance confirmation, 52

   remote access, 53–55

   security of patient records, 54–55

   Yellow Pages versus, 39–40

Internet Dental Directory, 40

Interruptions, 89–90

Interviewing prospective employees, 23–25

Inventory, maintaining, 70

J

Johnson, Spencer, 125

L

Laboratory, 74

Laughter, 107

Leadership skills, 27–29

Leasing equipment and facilities, 70

Leisure, 106

Lifelong learning, 123

Limited liability company (LLC), 15

Limited liability partnership (LLP), 15

M

Mahrabian, Dr. Albert, 119

Malpractice insurance, 70, 121

Managed care cost assessment, 65

Management
  business plan component, 11–12
  office manager, 28

Marital status, 25

Marketing, 31–40
  budget, 35–36, 134
  evaluating, 38–40
  hospital, relationship with, 12
  internal, 37–38
  outline, 10
  referrals, 31–33

Medco Health Solutions, 58

Media control, security, 54

Medical Economics, 78

Medical Group Management Association
  benefits of joining, 28–29
  pay ranges, 19
  revenue per patient, 17

Medicare
  antikickback statute, 75–76
  clinical lab services, 75
  e-prescribing, 57–58

Medicare and Medicaid Patient Protection Act of 1987, 75–76

Medication. *See* Prescriptions

Meditation, 106

Miami Children's Hospital mission statement, 2

Mission statement
  marketing plan, 35
  writing, 1–3

Multitasking, 90

N

Narcotics, 60

National Association of Chain Drug Stores (NACDS), 58

National Community Pharmacists Association (NCPA), 58

National ePrescribing Patient Safety Initiative (NEPSI), 58–59

National origin, 25

Noncompliant patients, 81–82, 120–122

Non-medical malpractice insurance coverage, 97–100

Note-takers, 90

O

Office design, 101–103
    benchmarks and equations, 133
    internal marketing, 37
    overhead, controlling, 70
Office dynamics, 45–46
Office location, 5–8
Office manager, 28
Office manual, 41–43
One Minute For Yourself (Johnson), 125
Online billing and insurance confirmation, 52
Operations policy manual, 41–43
Ornstein, Hal, mission statement, 3
Overhead costs, 69–71
Overhead expense assessment, 65
Ownership, 48–49
Owning office space, pros and cons, 7

P

Paperless office. *See* computer usage
Paperwork, 90, 110
Partners, adding, 93–96
A Passion for Excellence (Peters), 49
Patients
    budgeting, 17–18
    can't pay, 114–115
    communication and compliance, 81–83
    don't pay, 113–114
    encounter assessments, 65
    e-prescribing, 59
    getting referrals, 31–33
    importance of focusing on, 45–46
    per visit calculations, 17–18
    reviewing marketing efforts, 38
    scheduling, 109–111
    selling products to, 77–78
    won't pay, 115
Payroll ratio, 22, 66–67, 134
Per patient revenue average, 133
Personal and professional lives, balancing, 123–125
Personal health record (PHR), 52
Personal questions, 25
Person authentication, 55
Per visit value (PVV), 66, 134
Peters, Tom, 49

Physician Office Managers Association of America, 29

Prescriptions

    controlled substances, 60

    e-prescribing, 52, 57–60

    selling, 77–78

Prioritizing, 46, 92

Privacy, office design, 102

Product assessment, 66

Products, selling, 77–79

Professional corporation (PC), 15

Professional organizations

    benchmarks, 67–68, 133–135

    for staff, 28–29

Property coverage insurance, 97

Protocols, 46, 95–96

Q

QxMD, 54

R

Receptionist, 51

Reception room

    check-in and check-out areas, 102

    size, 102

    space requirements, 8

Referrals

    obtaining from doctors, 31–33

    recording from patients, 38–39

Reframing viewpoints to reduce stress, 106–107

Relaxation, 106

Religious life, 107

Remote access computer programs, 53–55

Renting office space, pros and cons, 6–7

Resignation procedures, 42

Respect, 48–49, 120

Responsiblity, 48–49

Return on investment (ROI), ancillary services, 75

Revenue leakage, 85–87

Risk management security, 100

S

Safety procedures, 42

Salary, associates, 94–95

Same-day patients, 109–110

Schedule

appointments, making online, 51

    mastering, 89

    planning, 45

Schwartz, Dr. Daniel, 54

S corp, 16

Scribes, 90

Security

    Internet records, 54–55

    property surveillance, 100

Selling products, 77–79

Service assessment, 66

Services

    ancillary, 73–76

    overhead, 70

Skyscape, Inc., 54

Sleep, 106

Smartphones, 53

Snell & Wilmer LLP Law Offices mission statement, 2

Sole proprietorship, 15

Space needs, office, 7–8, 102–103

Spiritual life, 107

Spouse, hiring for office staff, 22–23

Staff. *See also* Associates

    benchmark, 134

    benefits, 19–20, 41–42

    delegating responsibility, 91–92

    expenses, breaking down, 69

    hiring, 21–25

    motivation, 47–49

    office dynamics, 45–46

    office manager, 28

    office manual, 41–43

    overhead, asking for ways to reduce, 19–20, 71

    pay range, 18–19

    payroll ratio, 66–67

    professional organizations, 28–29

    security issues, 100

    time management, 89

Stark Law, 75

Stress management, 105–107

Stylish office design, 101

Suicide rates among doctors, 105

Support system, 107

SureScripts-RxHub, 58

Surveillance system, 100

T

Tablet computers, 53

Target, 110

Target, mission statement as, 1–2

Telephone

    collecting bills, 114

    online appointment scheduling, 51

    relationship with patients, 83

    services, cutting costs, 70

Termination procedures, 42

Third-party payers, 13–14

Time blocks, 109

Time management, 89–92

Time-outs, 106

Tracking Internet use, 40

Training employees, 23

Transmission security, 55

Travel time, 5

Treatment rooms, size of, 102

Trends, tracking, 67

Two-by-Four Rule, 82

U

Unrealistic expectations, 106

UPOD (Under-Promise and Over-Deliver), 82

US Department of Health and Human Services (DHHS), 52

W

The Walt Disney Company mission statement, 3

Web site, appointment scheduling by, 51

Woods, Dr. Michael, 121

Work culture, office manual and, 41

Workers' compensation, 98

Workflow study, 90–91

Work/life balance, achieving, 123–125

Y

Yellow Pages, 39–40